# Handbook of Prehospital Medications

*Emergency Care in the Streets*

# Handbook of Prehospital Medications

---

**Nancy L. Caroline, M.D.**

Adjunct Professor of Anesthesiology/Critical Care Medicine
University of Pittsburgh School of Medicine
Pittsburgh, Pennsylvania

Little, Brown and Company
Boston New York Toronto London

First Edition



Library of Congress Cataloging-in-Publication Data

Caroline, Nancy L.
Handbook of prehospital medications / Nancy L. Caroline.
p. cm.
Includes bibliographical references and index.
ISBN 0-316-55447-2
1. Drugs—Handbooks, manuals, etc. 2. Emergency medical technicians—Handbooks, manuals, etc. I. Title.
[DNLM: 1. Drug Therapy—handbooks. 2. Emergency Medicine—handbooks. 3. Drugs—administration & dosage—handbooks. 4. Drug—contraindications—handbooks.
WB 39 C292h 1995]
RM300.C37 1995
615.5′8—dc20
DNLM/DLC
for Library of Congress 94-32684
CIP

Printed in the United States of America

RRD-VA

Editorial: Evan R. Schnittman
Production Editor: Marie A. Salter
Copyeditor: Debra Corman
Production Supervisor/Designer: Cate Rickard

To Dr. Alexander Waller

# Contents

# Preface

Not every piece of information you learn in a paramedic course is worth storing forever in your head. And even some of the information that *is* worth storing in your head isn't always so easy to retrieve from memory when you need it, especially at 4 o'clock in the morning toward the end of a busy shift. But busy shift or not, there are some things you just have to get right. Medication information is one of those things. Forgetting a contraindication to a drug or getting the dosage wrong can have fatal consequences.

Just about all of the information a paramedic needs to safely administer the drugs most commonly used in the field is contained in *Emergency Care in the Streets* (Little, Brown, 1995). But weighing in at nearly 5 pounds (2.25 kilograms), *Emergency Care in the Streets* isn't very handy to carry around to every emergency. For that reason, we've taken all of the critical drug information that appears in that textbook (and some bonus information that does not appear there) and put it into a compact form that a paramedic can easily stash in a pocket or jump kit. So when you need to recheck a dosage in a hurry, or to make sure that the drug the physician ordered is not contraindicated in the particular case you're treating, you'll have a quick reference book right at your fingertips.

This handbook provides a variety of useful information about the drugs you use in the field and those that your patients may be taking at home. A list of commonly used **abbreviations** is provided to help you sort out the code in which doctors write prescriptions and order medicines. There is a chart to remind you of the classes of **drugs affecting the autonomic nervous system.** Formulas are given to help **calculate drug dosages and infusion rates,** both for adults and children. Separate tables list the **adult and pediatric dosages of commonly used drugs.** For each of 45 medications that may be used in the field, a **de-**

**tailed drug summary** is provided in standard format, so that you can find what you are looking for in a hurry. **Blank drug summary pages** are furnished to enable you to fill in information about any drugs introduced in your service that are not mentioned in this handbook. Finally, two extensive lists of **commonly prescribed drugs** are included—one organized alphabetically by trade name, the other by generic name—to help you identify the medications your patients are taking at home and to help you make some intelligent guesses, from that information, about the nature of patients' underlying illnesses.

Administering medications is one of the tasks that distinguishes a paramedic from an EMT-A. We have prepared this handbook with the hope of making that task a little safer and easier.

N.L.C.

# Handbook of Prehospital Medications

**Notice**

The indications and dosages of all drugs in this book have been recommended in the medical literature and conform to the practices of the general medical community. The medications described do not necessarily have specific approval by the Food and Drug Administration for use in the diseases and dosages for which they are recommended. The package insert for each drug should be consulted for use and dosage as approved by the FDA. Because standards for usage change, it is advisable to keep abreast of revised recommendations, particularly those concerning new drugs.

# Commonly Used Abbreviations Relating to Medications

| Abbreviation | Meaning |
|---|---|
| **ac** | Before meals |
| **amp** | Ampule |
| **ad lib** | As much as desired |
| **bid** | Twice a day |
| **c** | With |
| **caps** | Capsule |
| **cc** | Cubic centimeter (= 1 milliliter) |
| **D/C** | Discontinue |
| **D5/W** | 5% dextrose in water |
| **g** or **gm** | Gram |
| **gtt** | Drop |
| **h** or **hr** | Hour |
| **hs** | At bedtime |
| **IC** | Intracardiac |
| **IM** | Intramuscular |
| **IO** | Intraosseous |
| **IV** | Intravenous |
| **kg** | Kilogram (= 1,000 grams) |
| **L** | Liter (= 1,000 milliliters) |
| **LR(S)** | Lactated Ringer's solution |
| **mEq** | Milliequivalent |
| **mg** | Milligram |
| **μg** | Microgram |
| **ml** | Milliliter (= 1/1,000 liter) |
| **NG** | Nasogastric |
| **$N_2O$** | Nitrous oxide |
| **NPO** | Nothing by mouth |
| **NS** | Normal saline |
| **NTG** | Nitroglycerin |
| **OD** | Overdose |
| **$O_2$** | Oxygen |
| **p** | After |
| **pc** | After meals |
| **PO** | By mouth |
| **PR** | Per rectum |
| **prn** | As needed |
| **q** | Every |
| **q6h** | Every 6 hours |
| **qid** | Four times a day |
| **Rx** | Prescription, treatment |
| **s** | Without |
| **SC** or **SQ** | Subcutaneous |
| **SL** | Sublingual |
| **stat** | Immediately |
| **tab** | Tablet |
| **tid** | Three times a day |
| **TKVO** | To keep vein open |

# Autonomic Drugs: Summary

| Features | Parasympathetic System | Sympathetic System: Alpha ($\alpha$) | Sympathetic System: Beta ($\beta$) |
|---|---|---|---|
| Other name | Cholinergic | Adrenergic | |
| Natural chemical mediator | Acetylcholine (ACh) | Norepinephrine (chiefly alpha) | Epinephrine (chiefly beta) |
| Primary nerve(s) | Vagus | Nerves from the thoracic and lumbar ganglia of the spinal cord | |
| Effect of stimulation | Slows the heart<br>Constricts pupils<br>Increases salivation<br>Increases gut motility | Constricts blood vessels<br>Slows the gut<br>Dilates pupils | Dilates blood vessels<br>Speeds heart ($\beta_1$)<br>Dilates bronchi ($\beta_2$) |
| Stimulating drug | Neostigmine<br>Reserpine | Phenylephrine<br>**Dopamine** (high dose)<br>**Norepinephrine***<br>Metaraminol* | Isoproterenol<br>**Albuterol** ($\beta_2$)<br>**Isoetharine** ($\beta_2$)<br>**Terbutaline** ($\beta_2$)<br>**Epinephrine***<br>**Dopamine** (low dose)<br>**Dobutamine** ($\beta_1$) |
| Blocking drugs | **Atropine** | Chlorpromazine<br>Phentolamine | **Propranolol**<br>**Labetalol**<br>Atenolol |

Mixed alpha and beta effects.

# Drug Dosage Calculations

- Calculation of **drug concentration** in an ampule of vial:

  **Concentration = total mg/total ml**

- Calculation of **drug concentration** when drug is described **as a percentage** (e.g., 25% magnesium sulfate or 1% lidocaine):

  **% = grams/100 ml,** therefore:

  1. **grams/100 ml × 1,000 = milligrams/100 ml**
  2. **milligrams/100 ml ÷ 100 = mg/ml**

- Calculation of **dosage** for drugs labeled in mg/ml:

  $$\textbf{Volume to be administered} = \frac{\textbf{desired dose (mg)}}{\textbf{concentration on hand (mg/ml)}}$$

- Calculation of **IV drug infusion rate:**

  1. Calculate **desired dose (mg or μg) per minute:**

     **Desired dose/min = dose/kg/min × patient's weight (kg)**

  2. Calculate flow rate in **ml/min**:

     $$\textbf{Flow rate (ml/min)} = \frac{\textbf{desired dose (mg/min or μg/min)}}{\textbf{concentration of infusion (mg/ml or μg/ml)}}$$

  3. Calculate the **drip rate**:

     **Drip rate (drops/min) = flow rate (ml/min) × drops/ml**

*Note:* Microdrip tubing delivers 60 drops/ml.

# Calculating Pediatric Dosages

Most pediatric drug dosages are based on the child's weight in kilograms. If you are given the child's weight in pounds, therefore, you must convert it to kilograms:

$$\textbf{Weight in kilograms} = \frac{\textbf{Weight in pounds}}{\textbf{2.2}}$$

If you do not carry a scale in the ambulance and the parent cannot tell you the child's weight, you can obtain a rough estimate of the weight from the following chart:

**AGE-RELATED WEIGHTS IN CHILDREN**

| Age | Weight (kg) |
|---|---|
| Newborn | 3–5 |
| 1 year | 10 |
| 3 years | 15 |
| 5 years | 20 |
| 8 years | 25 |
| 10 years | 30 |
| 15 years | 50 |

If you misplace your weight chart, you can use the following equation as a rough guide to calculate the weight of a child up to age 9:

$$\textbf{Weight (kg)} = (\textbf{Age [in years]} \times 2) + 9$$

# Prehospital Medications: Pediatric Dosages

| Drug | Dosage | Route/Method |
|---|---|---|
| Activated charcoal | <12 yr: **15–30 gm**<br>>12 yr: **1 gm/kg** | **PO** (as a slurry in water)<br>**PO** (as a slurry in water) |
| Adenosine | **0.1–0.2 mg/kg/dose** | Rapid **IV** bolus |
| Aminophylline | **6 mg/kg** in 30 ml D5/W | **IV** infusion (30 min) |
| Atropine sulfate | *Cardiac arrest:* **0.02 mg/kg/dose** (minimum = 0.1 mg)<br>*Organophosphate poisoning:* **0.05 mg/kg/dose** | Slowly **IV** (30 sec)<br>**IV** (half the dose may be given IM) |
| 10% Calcium gluconate | **0.2 ml/kg** | Slowly **IV** (30 min) |
| 50% Dextrose | **0.5 gm/kg** diluted in equal volume of water for injection | Slowly **IV** through a large vein |
| Diazepam | **0.3 mg/kg**<br>**0.5 mg/kg** | **IV**<br>**Rectal** |
| Diphenhydramine | **1 mg/kg** | Slowly **IV** (5 min) |
| Dopamine | **2–20 µg/kg/min** | **IV** titrated infusion |
| Epinephrine | *Anaphylaxis:* **0.1 ml/kg of 1:10,000**<br>*Cardiac arrest:* 1st dose: **0.1 ml/kg of 1:10,000** (= 0.1 mg/kg) Next doses: 0.1 mg/kg<br>*Shock/bradycardia:* **0.1 µg/kg/min** | **IV** slow push<br>**IV** push or **endotracheal**<br>**IV** infusion |
| Furosemide | **1 mg/kg** | Slow **IV** push |
| Hydrocortisone | **7 mg/kg** | Slowly **IV** |
| Ipecac, syrup of | 6–9 mo: **5 ml,** then water<br>9–12 mo: **10 ml,** then water<br>1–12 yr: **15 ml,** then water<br>>12 yr: **30 ml,** then water | **PO**<br>**PO**<br>**PO**<br>**PO** |
| Isoetharine | **0.01 ml/kg** in 3 ml NS | **Inhalation** |
| Lidocaine | **1 mg/kg**<br>**20–50 µg/kg/min** | Slow **IV** push<br>**IV** infusion |
| Mannitol | **0.5 gm/kg** | Slow **IV** injection |
| Methylprednisolone | **1 mg/kg** | Slow **IV** push (5 min) |
| Morphine sulfate | **0.1 mg/kg** | Slow **IV** push |
| Naloxone | **0.01 mg/kg** (→ 0.1 mg/kg[a] → 0.2 mg/kg[b]) | Slow **IV** push |
| Sodium bicarbonate | **1 mEq/kg** | Slow **IV** push |
| Terbutaline | **0.03 ml/kg** in 3 ml NS<br>**0.01 mg/kg** | **Inhalation**<br>**SQ** |

[a] = 2nd dose.
[b] = 3rd dose.

# Drawing Up and Administering Drugs

**Guidelines for Administering Drugs in the Field**

- Make sure the physician at medical command understands the situation.
- Make sure *you* understand the physician's orders clearly. **When in doubt, ask** the physician to repeat the order.
- Always **repeat orders back** to the physician before administering a medication, to confirm that you received the order accurately.
- Confirm that the patient is **not allergic** to the medication that has been ordered (ask the patient or a family member; look for a medical identification tag).
- **Read the drug label carefully** as you take the vial or syringe from its box and again before you give the drug. Make a note of the **drug concentration** printed on the label and the drug's **date of expiration.**
- **Check for defects** in the vial or ampule, and make sure that the fluid inside is not cloudy, discolored, or precipitated. If the medication is in any way suspect, do *not* use it.
- If you have orders to administer more than one drug, **make sure that the drugs are not incompatible.**
- Notify the physician at medical command when the drug has been administered.
- **Monitor the patient** for possible adverse side effects.
- **Dispose of the syringe and needle safely.** Do *not* try to recap the needle.

## *Using a Tubex System*

A Tubex system consists of a stainless steel housing and a prefilled, disposable cartridge (*A*). The system is used most often for the injection of controlled substances, such as morphine. To assemble a Tubex syringe:

1. Swing the plunger handle of the syringe down (*B*).
2. **Check the label** on the cartridge to make sure it is the drug you want to give and to determine the concentration.
3. Insert the cartridge into the cartridge housing (*C*).
4. Screw the cartridge into the housing (*D*).
5. Bring the plunger back into alignment with the cartridge housing, and screw it into the cartridge (*E*).
6. Expel any air from the dead space in the cartridge (*F*).

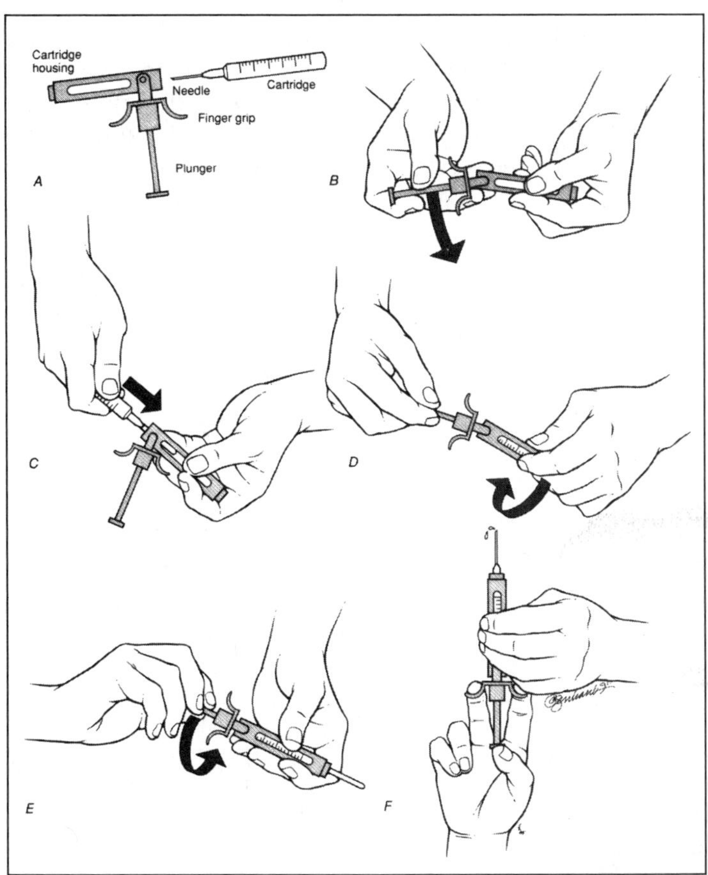

## *Using a Prefilled Syringe*

A prefilled syringe is supplied as a plastic barrel/needle assembly and a glass cartridge containing the medication. To use a prefilled syringe:

1. **Check the label** on the cartridge to make certain it is the drug you want.
2. **Inspect** the contents of the cartridge for discoloration, cloudiness, or particulate matter. (If any of those is present, discard the cartridge and take another.)
3. **Pop off the caps** from both the medication cartridge and the plastic barrel (*A*).
4. **Insert the cartridge** into the barrel, and twist it into place (*B*).
5. Hold the cartridge with the needle pointing up, and tap on it to bring any air inside it to the top (*C*). Then briefly uncap the needle, **expel the air,** and—if you do not intend to inject the contents of the cartridge immediately—*carefully* recap the needle.

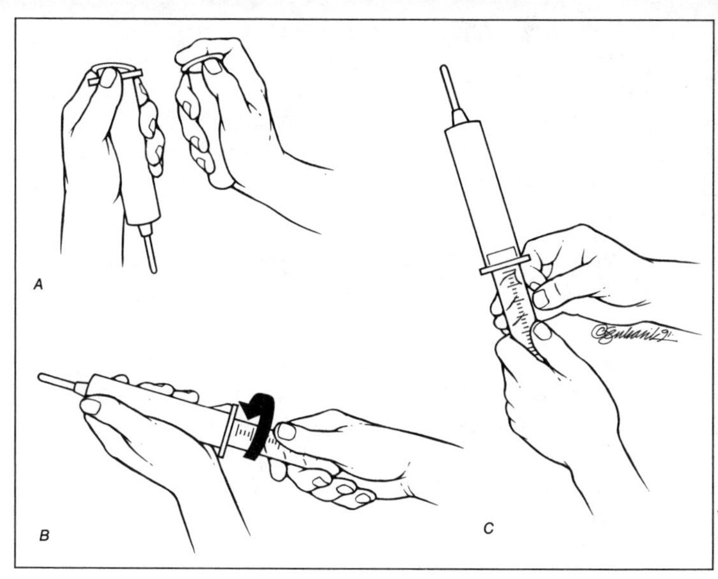
A
B
C

## *Drawing Up a Drug from an Ampule*

An **ampule** is a glass container in which a *single dose* of a sterile drug preparation is sealed. Ampules are used to store drugs given by injection, such as epinephrine or furosemide. To draw up medication from an ampule into a syringe, proceed as follows:

1. **Prepare a syringe** of the appropriate volume with a needle of the appropriate gauge, depending on whether you will be giving the medication IV, IM, or SQ.
2. Read the **name and concentration** of the medication printed on the ampule to confirm that you have the right drug and concentration.
3. **Inspect** the solution for discoloration, cloudiness, or particles (*A*). Do not use a solution that is discolored, cloudy, or has particulate matter in it.
4. **Compute the volume** of the drug you need to draw up (see p. 3 for the formula for computing drug volume).
5. Snap your finger sharply against the stem of the ampule (*B*) to move the solution down into the well of the ampule.
6. If the ampule does not have a colored band around the stem, you will have to score its stem with the small metal file supplied with the ampule. If the ampule does have a colored circle around the stem, it will break cleanly without being scored.
7. Grasp the top of the ampule in a 4-by-4-inch gauze pad, to protect your fingers from injury, and **break off the top** of the ampule at the stem (*C*).
8. **Insert the needle** into the ampule, taking care that the needle does not touch the ampule's rim.
9. Pull back on the plunger of the syringe (*D*) to **draw up the specified volume** of medication, according to the dosage you calculated.
10. **Expel any air** present in the syringe (*E*), and—if you are not planning to inject the medication immediately—*carefully* recap the needle.

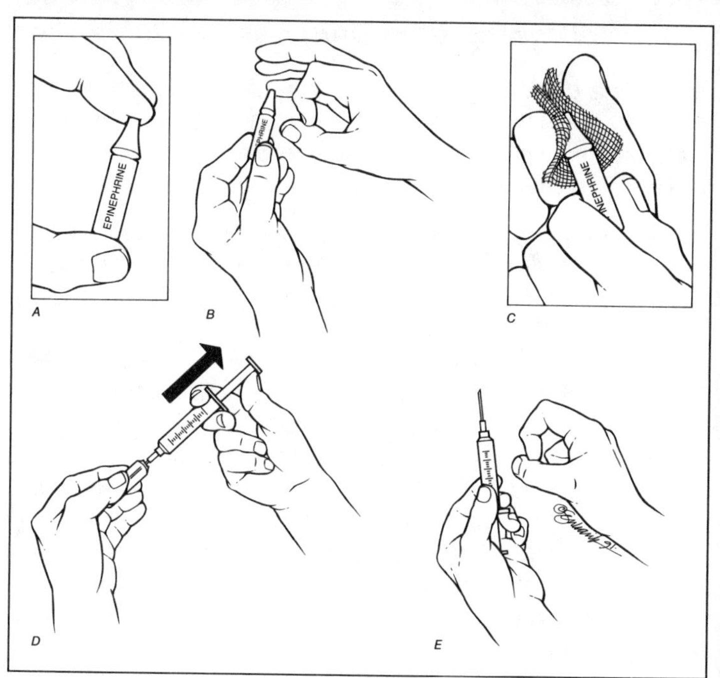
EPINEPHRINE
EPHRINE
NEPHRINE
A
B
C
D
E

## *Drawing Up a Drug from a Vial*

A **vial** is a glass container storing sterile powdered or liquid drugs for parenteral use. It differs from an ampule in that a vial is sealed with a rubber stopper and may contain *multiple doses.* To draw up a solution from a vial:

1. **Prepare a syringe** of the appropriate volume with a needle of the appropriate gauge (according to whether you are going to give the medication IV, IM, or SQ).
2. Read the **name and concentration of the medication** printed on the vial to confirm that you are using the medication ordered.
3. **Inspect the solution** for discoloration, cloudiness, or particles. Do not use a solution that is discolored, cloudy, or has particulate matter in it.
4. **Compute the volume** of the drug you need to draw up (see formulas on p. 3).
5. **Disinfect** the rubber stopper of the vial with an alcohol swab.
6. **Draw air into the syringe** in a volume equal to that of the solution to be withdrawn.
7. **Insert the needle** at an angle through the rubber stopper of the vial, and **inject** the **air** into the vial (see figure).
8. With the vial inverted, **draw up the specified volume** of medication according to the dosage you calculated.
9. **Withdraw** the needle from the vial.
10. Expel any air present in the syringe, and—if you are not going to inject the contents of the syringe immediately—*carefully* recap the needle.

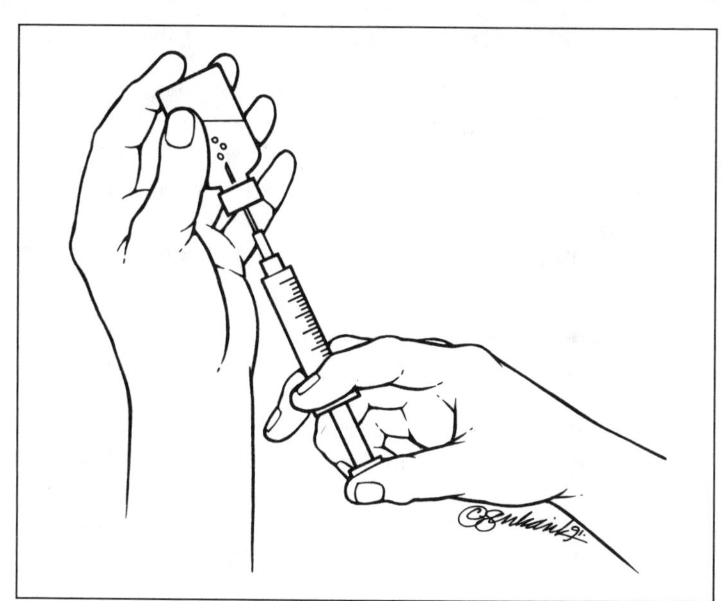

## *Giving Drugs Through an IV Line*

When ordered to give a medication by "IV push," it is preferable to do so through an established intravenous line rather than directly into a vein, because the chances of the drug infiltrating are greater if you are trying to hold a needle steady inside a vein while pushing on the plunger of the syringe. The procedure for injecting a medication through an IV line is as follows:

1. **Disinfect** the drug administration port on the IV line with an alcohol swab (*A*).
2. **Uncap the needle** from your syringe.
3. **Insert the needle** into the drug administration port, taking care not to jam it straight through and out the other side!
4. **Pinch the tubing** distal to the port (i.e., farther from the patient) to prevent the drug from flowing backward into the IV bag.
5. **Inject** the medication *slowly* (*B*).
6. **Withdraw the needle** from the port, and dispose of the needle and syringe in a safe receptacle.
7. **Open the control clamp** wide to flush any remaining medication from the line (*C*).
8. **Readjust the clamp** so that the IV is running at the rate ordered.
9. **Monitor** the patient carefully for signs of an adverse reaction to the drug.

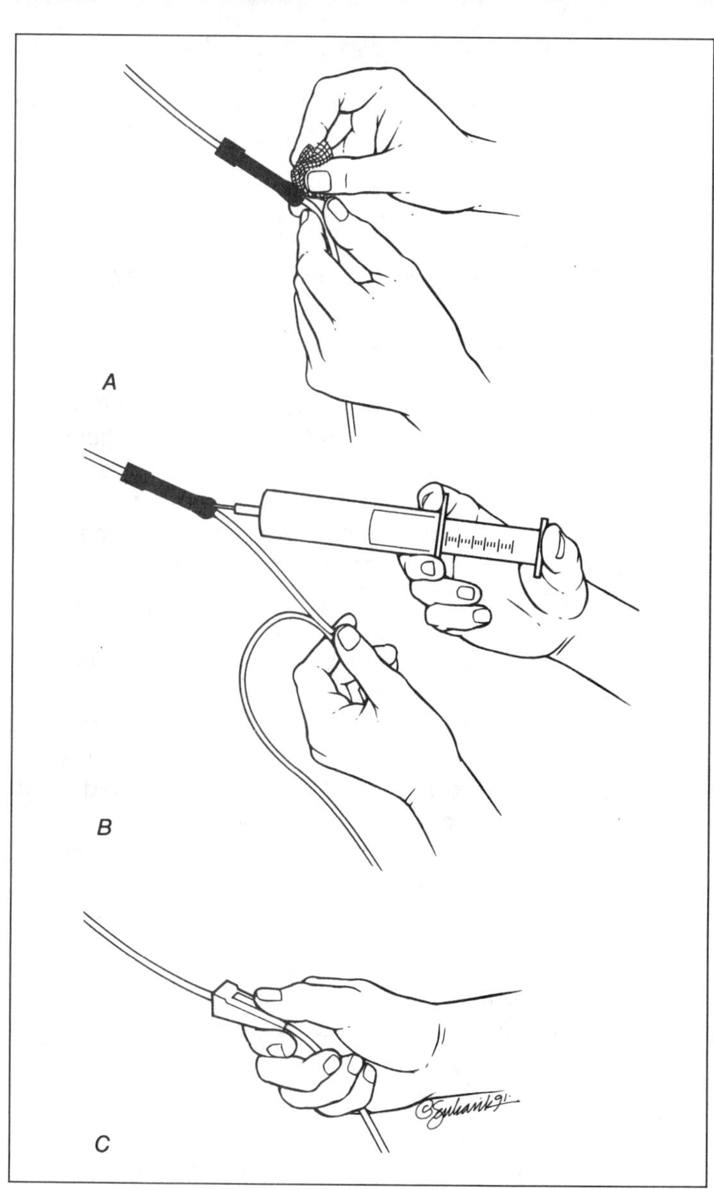
A
B
C
©Sykarik 91

## *Adding Drugs to an IV Bag*

Drugs whose effects must be carefully titrated, such as dopamine or norepinephrine, are added to the intravenous solution rather than administered directly to the patient:

1. **Set up the IV** bag and administration set in the usual manner.
2. **Check the drug name** on the vial, ampule, or prefilled syringe.
3. **Check the concentration** of the drug in the vial, ampule, or prefilled syringe.
4. **Compute the volume** of drug to be added to the IV bag (see p. 3 for the formula for computing intravenous drug dosages).
5. **Draw up** in a syringe the volume you calculated (if a prefilled syringe is used, note what proportion of the volume of the syringe is required).
6. **Close the control clamp** on the administration set (*A*).
7. **Disinfect** the rubber stopper or sleeve on the IV bag with an alcohol swab.
8. **Puncture** the stopper with the needle, and inject the desired volume of medication into the IV bag (*B*).
9. **Withdraw the needle,** and discard the needle and syringe in an appropriate container.
10. **Agitate the IV bag** gently to be sure that the added drug is well mixed into the solution.
11. **Label** the bag with
    - **Name of the medication** added.
    - **Amount** added.
    - **Resulting concentration** of medication in the bag (in mg/ml or µg/ml).
    - **Date and time.**
    - **Your name.**
12. **Calculate the rate** at which the IV must be run (drops/min) to deliver the desired dose of medication (see formulas on p. 3).

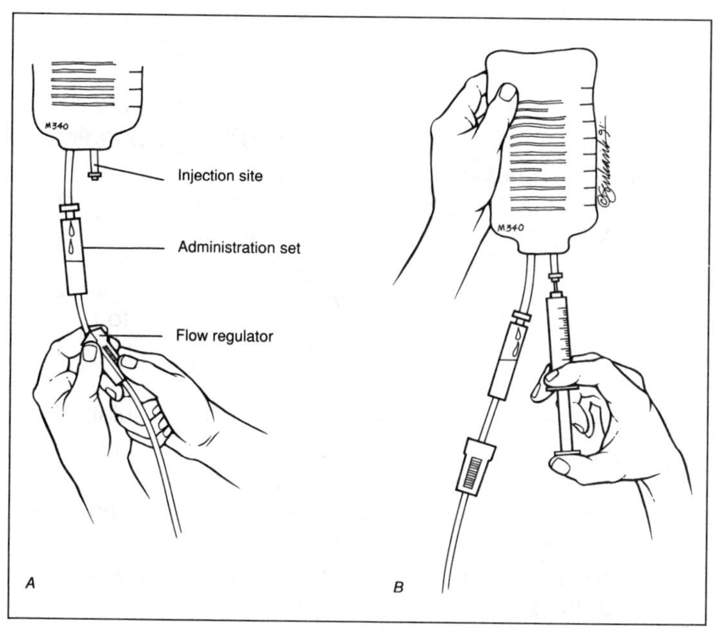
M340
Injection site
Administration set
Flow regulator
A
M340
B

## Giving an Intramuscular Injection

| AVOID IN | GIVEN FOR |
|---|---|
| Acute myocardial infarction<br>Any condition of poor peripheral perfusion (e.g., shock) | Uncomplicated fractures with long transport times (pain relief)<br>Patients requiring thiamine (half the dose is usually given IM)<br>Patients with organophosphate poisoning (two-thirds of the atropine dose is given IM) |

**Procedure**

1. Explain the procedure to the patient, and **obtain consent.**
2. Verify that the patient is **not allergic** to the drug you plan to administer.
3. Prepare a **syringe (2–5 ml),** and attach a **21-gauge needle.**
4. **Check the label** on the medication container.
5. **Compute the dosage,** and **draw up** the desired volume in the syringe (see p. 3 for the formula for computing dosage).
6. Locate the **deltoid** muscle (*A*).
7. **Disinfect** the injection site with an alcohol swab (*B*).
8. With one hand, bunch the deltoid muscle together. Hold the syringe in your other hand like a dart, and **quickly thrust the needle** into the tissue at a **90-degree angle** (*C*).
9. **Pull back slightly on the plunger** of the syringe to be sure that the needle has not accidently entered a blood vessel (*D*).
10. If there is no blood return into the syringe, **inject** the medication (*E*). (*Note:* If there *is* blood return, withdraw the needle, hold pressure over the puncture site for a minute, then try again at another site.)

11. Quickly **withdraw** the needle, and apply firm pressure over the injection site with a sterile pad (*F*).
12. Dispose of the needle and syringe in an appropriate receptacle.
13. **Monitor** the patient for adverse reactions to the medication.

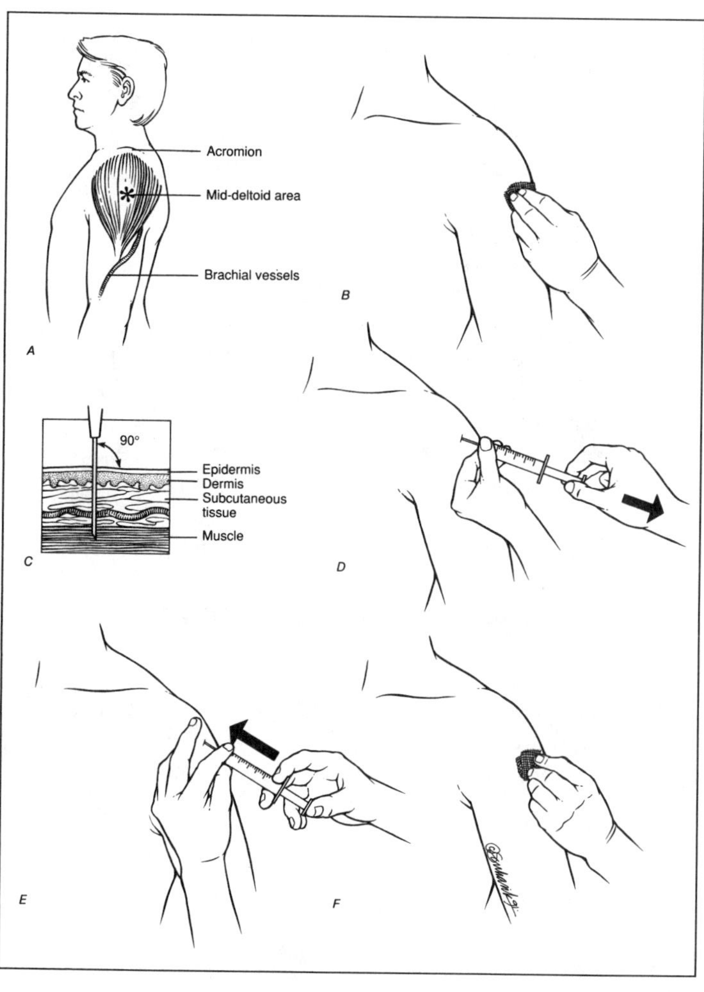

## *Giving a Subcutaneous Injection*

The subcutaneous route is used in prehospital care chiefly for the administration of terbutaline to patients with severe asthma or of epinephrine to patients with moderate anaphylaxis. The technique is as follows:

1. **Explain** the procedure to the patient, and **obtain consent.**
2. Verify that the patient is **not allergic** to the drug you plan to administer.
3. Prepare a **1-ml syringe,** and attach a **25-gauge needle.**
4. **Check the label** on the medication container to verify the drug name and concentration.
5. **Compute the dosage,** and draw up the desired volume in the syringe (see p. 3 for formula for computing dosage).
6. Locate the **deltoid** muscle.
7. **Disinfect** the injection site with an alcohol swab.
8. Gently grasp the skin over the injection site, and pull it away from the overlying muscle. **Insert the needle** into the subcutaneous tissue at a **45-degree angle** to the skin (see figure).
9. **Pull back slightly on the plunger** to be sure that the needle has not accidentally entered a blood vessel.
10. If there is no blood return into the syringe, **inject** the medication.
11. Quickly **withdraw** the needle, at the same angle as it was inserted, and apply firm pressure over the injection site.
12. Dispose of the needle and syringe in an appropriate receptacle.
13. **Monitor** the patient for adverse reactions to the medication.

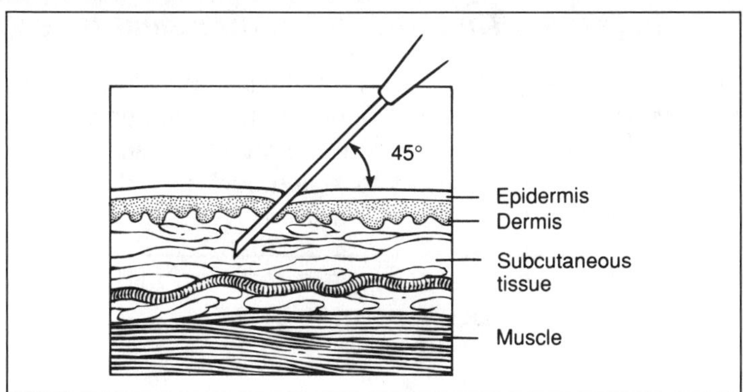
45°
Epidermis
Dermis
Subcutaneous
tissue
Muscle

## *Giving Drugs Through an Endotracheal Tube*

The endotracheal route is used when it is impossible to start a reliable intravenous line. Among the medications used in prehospital care, only a few may be given by the endotracheal route. The easiest way to remember which drugs may be given endotracheally is by the word "NAVEL":

| DRUGS THAT MAY BE GIVEN VIA AN ENDOTRACHEAL TUBE | |
|---|---|
| **N** | naloxone |
| **A** | atropine |
| **V** | Valium (diazepam) |
| **E** | epinephrine |
| **L** | lidocaine |

Absorption from the tracheobronchial tree is nearly as rapid as absorption from an intravenous injection. In most cases, when you give a drug via the endotracheal tube, you will need to use 2 to 2.5 times the intravenous dosage. The procedure is as follows:

1. While someone else ventilates the patient, **dilute the required dose** of the medication in a syringe containing **10 ml of sterile water.**
2. **Disconnect** the bag-valve device from the endotracheal tube, and rapidly **squirt** the contents of the syringe down the tube (*A*).
3. Immediately **reconnect** the bag to the endotracheal tube, and **ventilate** the patient briskly to facilitate passage of the medication down the trachea (*B*).

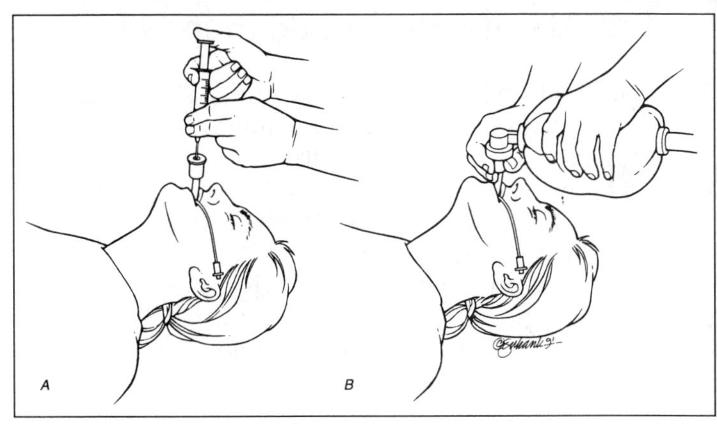
A
B

# Profiles of Drugs Used in the Field

This section of the handbook contains a detailed description of the majority of drugs used by paramedic services in the United States. The first page of this section illustrates the general format in which each drug will be presented. There follows detailed information on 45 medications, **listed alphabetically by generic name.**

Following the drug profiles, we have provided some **blank pages in the same format,** so that you can fill in information about any new drugs introduced into your service that are not covered in this handbook.

# Format for Drug Information

For each drug presented in this section, you will find the following information:

| **Generic Name**<br><br>Trade Name(s) |
|---|
| **Therapeutic Effects**<br>What **class** of drug is it? What is its **mechanism of action?** What is the **desired effect** that giving the drug is supposed to produce? |
| **Indications**<br>For what **medical conditions** is the drug usually given? |
| **Contraindications**<br>Under what conditions should the drug *not* be administered? |
| **Side Effects**<br>What predictable effects, especially **undesirable effects** (e.g., nausea, hypotension), occur in addition to the therapeutic effects when the drug is administered? |
| **How Supplied**<br>In what **form** is the drug supplied (in tablets? in ampules? in vials? in prefilled syringes?), in what **volume,** and what is the **concentration** (usually given in mg/ml) of the drug as it is supplied by the manufacturer? |
| **Administration and Dosage**<br>By what **route(s)** is the drug usually given? What is the usual **dosage** for each route? What is the correct **timing** of administration (by rapid IV bolus? by slow IV push? by infusion at a certain rate?)? If the drug needs to be diluted for a titrated intravenous infusion, how much drug should be diluted into what volume of diluent and what is the **final concentration** after dilution? |
| **Incompatibility**<br>Is the drug incompatible with any other medication that you might give or that the patient might be taking at home? |

# Activated Charcoal USP

Charcodote, SuperChar

**Therapeutic Effects**
Adsorbs many poisonous compounds to its surface, thereby reducing their absorption by the body. Partially effective in binding aspirin, amphetamines, strychnine, phenytoin, theophylline, and phenobarbital.

**Indications**
Certain cases of **poisoning** and **overdose.**

**Contraindications**
No absolute contraindications, but not worthwhile or potentially hazardous in

- Poisoning due to *methanol, caustic acids and alkalis, iron tablets, lithium.*
- *Cyanide poisoning.*

Do not use if the container in which charcoal was stored has not been tightly sealed.

**Side Effects**
No serious adverse side effects.

**How Supplied**
Fine black powder in bottles of 25 gm and 50 gm.

**Administration and Dosage**
Given by mouth or through a nasogastric tube.

*Dosage:* A good rule of thumb for both children and adults is **1 gm/kg.** The charcoal is **mixed in tap water** to make a slurry.

**Incompatibility**
None.

Does *not* interfere with the action of syrup of ipecac or *N*-acetylcysteine.

# Adenosine

Adenocard

**Therapeutic Effects**

Slows discharge of the sinoatrial node and **delays conduction through the atrioventricular (AV) node.** Metabolized rapidly, so has a very short half-life ($<$10 sec) and its effects are very brief.

**Indications**

- First-line drug for narrow-complex **paroxysmal supraventricular tachycardia** (PSVT).
- May be used diagnostically (*after* lidocaine) in wide-complex tachycardia of uncertain type.

**Contraindications**

- **Second- or third-degree AV block.**
- Sick sinus syndrome.
- Patients taking **incompatible drugs** (see below).

**Side Effects**

Very common, but transient. The following side effects usually resolve by themselves within 1 to 2 minutes:

- **Flushing.**
- **Dyspnea.**
- **Chest pain** or tightness.
- **Headache.**

In addition, adenosine often causes **brief cardiac dysrhythmias** immediately after conversion of PSVT, especially

- Sinus bradycardia and even brief asystole.
- Premature ventricular contractions (PVCs).

Because adenosine has a short half-life, **PSVT may recur.**

**How Supplied**

In vials containing 6 mg in 2 ml. (The vials should not be refrigerated, as the solution may crystallize in cold temperatures.)

# Adenosine (continued)

## Administration and Dosage

The patient should be **recumbent** with the stretcher tilted slightly **head-up.**

Adenosine is given through the IV line at the *most proximal injection port:*

- Initial dosage: **6 mg by rapid IV bolus** over 1 to 3 seconds, followed immediately by **20 ml of saline** to flush the drug into the circulation.
- If there is no response within 1 to 2 minutes, a **repeat dose of 12 mg by rapid IV bolus** may be given.
- A third dose, of 12 mg, may be given after 1 to 2 minutes if needed.
- If PSVT is corrected by adenosine but then keeps recurring, try verapamil or propranolol.

## Incompatibility

Do not give adenosine to patients taking either **dipyridamole** (Persantine) or **carbamazepine** (Tegretol), both of which prolong and potentiate adenosine's effects.

Adenosine is *less effective* in patients taking *theophylline* preparations (which many asthmatics use) or other xanthines such as *coffee.*

# Albuterol/Salbutamol

Proventil, Ventolin

**Therapeutic Effects**

Selective **beta-2** sympathomimetic drug, that is, a beta agent that acts primarily on the *bronchial* musculature rather than the myocardium. Therefore, albuterol relaxes bronchial smooth muscle and **relieves bronchospasm.**

**Indications**

Drug of *first choice* for relief of bronchospasm associated with **acute asthmatic attacks** or exacerbation of **chronic bronchitis.**

**Contraindications**

- **Tachyarrhythmias.**
- Use with *caution* in patients with **hypertension, angina,** or **diabetes.**

**Side Effects**

- Palpitations, tachycardia.
- Tremor, nervousness.
- Dizziness.
- Nausea, heartburn.

**How Supplied**

- Metered-dose inhaler.
- Bottles of 0.5% solution for use in nebulizer.

**Administration and Dosage**

If using a *metered-dose inhaler,* attach a spacer. The patient should take **1 to 2 inhalations.** The dose may be repeated in 15 minutes.

By *nebulizer:*

- *Dosage for adults and children over 12:* **Dilute** 0.5 ml of 0.5% solution **(2.5 mg**) in **3 ml of sterile saline,** and place that solution in the nebulizer. Regulate the flow rate of the nebulizer to deliver the 3 ml over **5 to 15 minutes.**
- *Pediatric dosage:* **0.01 to 0.03 mg/kg in 3 ml of sterile saline** via the nebulizer.

**Incompatibility**

May be ineffective in patients taking beta blockers (e.g., propranolol).

# Aminophylline

## Therapeutic Effects

Xanthine drug derived from theophylline with the following actions:

- Stimulation of the myocardium to increase heart rate and cardiac output.
- **Bronchodilation** and vasodilation (by smooth muscle relaxation).
- Strengthening of diaphragmatic contractions.
- Stimulation of respiratory drive.
- Increase in coronary blood flow.
- Mild diuretic.
- Central nervous system stimulation.

## Indications

A *second-line drug* for the following indications:

- For bronchodilation in acute attacks of **asthma** and in decompensated **chronic obstructive pulmonary disease** (COPD).
- To relieve bronchoconstriction in **anaphylaxis.**
- To relieve bronchoconstriction in selected cases of **congestive heart failure** and **pulmonary edema** from other causes.

## Contraindications

Relative contraindications:

- Cardiac **dysrhythmias,** especially tachyarrhythmias and premature ventricular contractions (PVCs).
- **Hypotension.**
- Massive **acute myocardial infarction.**

## Side Effects

- Myocardial irritability and **dysrhythmias,** especially in the presence of hypoxemia; palpitations.
- **Hypotension.**
- **Nausea** and **vomiting.**
- Headache.
- Excitement, confusion, **seizures.**

Because of the high risk of dangerous side effects, aminophylline is not a drug of first choice for any indication.

# **Aminophylline** (continued)

**How Supplied**

Ampules of 250 mg or 500 mg.

**Administration and Dosage**

Given **intravenously** through a peripheral IV line. For patients who are not already taking theophylline, start with a **bolus of 5 mg/kg in 50 ml of D5/W over 20 minutes;** follow with an infusion:

- For *acute asthmatic attacks:* Add 250 mg to 1 liter of D5/W, to make a solution of 0.25 mg/ml. **Infuse** at a rate of **0.5 mg/kg/hr.**
- For *pulmonary edema:* Add 250 mg to 250 ml of D5/W, to yield a solution of 1 mg/ml. **Infuse** at a rate of **0.5 mg/kg/hr.**

**Incompatibility**

Beta blockers may lessen effectiveness of aminophylline.

# Amyl Nitrite

Vaporole

**Therapeutic Effects**

- Oxidizes hemoglobin to methemoglobin, a form that competes with cytochrome oxidase for the cyanide ion; therefore helps inactivate the cyanide ion.
- Vasodilatation, including coronary artery dilatation (in the same family of drugs as nitroglycerin).
- As a smooth muscle relaxant, can relieve spasms of the biliary tract.

**Indications**

To treat **cyanide poisoning.**

**Contraindications**

**None** when used to treat cyanide poisoning.

**Side Effects**

- Marked **hypotension** due to sudden vasodilation, with syncope if the patient is not recumbent.
- Reflex **tachycardia** secondary to the drop in blood pressure.
- Cutaneous **flush** involving the head, neck, and clavicular regions.
- Pounding **headache.**
- Nausea and vomiting.

**How Supplied**

Perles (small ampules) of 0.2 to 0.3 ml.

**Administration and Dosage**

Start treatment *urgently* in suspected cyanide poisoning.

**Keep patient recumbent.** Break a perle into a gauze pad or handkerchief, hold it over the patient's face for **20 seconds,** then give **100% oxygen for 40 to 100 seconds.** Continue alternating amyl nitrite and 100% oxygen in that fashion all the way to the hospital.

**Incompatibility**

None of significance.

# Atropine Sulfate

**Therapeutic Effects**

By blocking parasympathetic (vagal) action of the heart, atropine

- Increases the rate of discharge by the sinoatrial (SA) node.
- Enhances conduction through the atrioventricular (AV) junction.

In addition to speeding up a slow heart to a normal rate, atropine reduces the chances of ectopic activity in the ventricles and thus of ventricular fibrillation. Most effective in **reversing bradycardia due to increased parasympathetic tone, morphine, or organophosphates;** less effective in treating bradycardias due to actual damage to the AV or SA node.

**Indications**

- **Sinus bradycardia** *when accompanied by premature ventricular contractions* (PVCs) *or hypotension.*
- **Type I second-degree AV block (Wenckebach)** when accompanied by bradycardia.
- Third-degree heart block when accompanied by symptomatic bradycardia in the context of *inferior*-wall acute myocardial infarction.
- In some cases of **asystole.**
- As an antidote in **organophosphate poisoning.**

**Contraindications**

None when used for life-threatening emergencies. Use with *caution* in patients with

- **Atrial flutter** or **atrial fibrillation** when there is a rapid ventricular response.
- **Type II second-degree AV block.**
- **Complete** (third-degree) **AV block** in the context of *anterior*-wall acute myocardial infarction.
- **Glaucoma.**
- **Chronic obstructive pulmonary disease.**

## Atropine Sulfate (continued)

### Side Effects

The patient should be warned that he or she may experience some of the following side effects and that these side effects are part of the drug's usual and expected actions:

- **Blurred vision, headache,** pupillary dilatation.
- **Dry mouth,** thirst.
- **Flushing** of the skin.
- Difficulty in urination (especially in older men).

Paradoxical **bradycardia** may occur if a dose less than 0.5 mg is given to an adult or if even the correct dose is given too slowly.

### How Supplied

Prefilled syringes in a variety of volumes and concentrations; *check the volume and concentration on every preloaded syringe before giving the drug!*
Ampules with 1 mg in 1 ml.
Multidose vials with a concentration of 1 mg/ml.

### Administration and Dosage

- For *bradycardia:* **0.5 to 1.0 mg IV,** repeated at 5-minute intervals until the desired heart rate is achieved; the *total dose should not exceed 2.0 mg.*
- For *organophosphate poisoning:* **2 mg IM and 1 mg IV.** The IV dose may be repeated every 5 to 10 minutes as needed, until a decrease in secretions is observed.
- For *asystole:* **1 mg IV or via endotracheal tube,** repeated in 5 minutes if asystole persists.

### Incompatibility

None of significance.

### Signs of Overdose or Toxicity

Mad as a hatter,
Hot as a hare,
Blind as a bat,
Red as a beet,
Dry as a bone.

# Bretylium Tosylate

Bretylol, Bretylate

**Therapeutic Effects**

- Raises the threshold of heart muscle for ventricular fibrillation.
- May reduce energy required for defibrillation.
- Occasionally converts ventricular fibrillation to an effective rhythm without electric countershock.

**Indications**

- **Ventricular fibrillation** that has not been successfully converted with countershock and lidocaine or that recurs despite lidocaine treatment.
- **Ventricular tachycardia** that has been unresponsive to first-line therapy (i.e., lidocaine and/or countershock).

**Contraindications**

None when used for life-threatening dysrhythmias.

**Side Effects**

- **Hypotension** (by beta blocking action); patients should be kept supine after receiving bretylium to minimize this effect.
- **Nausea** and **vomiting,** when the drug is given rapidly IV.

**How Supplied**

10-ml ampules containing 500 mg (50 mg/ml).

## Bretylium Tosylate (continued)

**Administration and Dosage**

Given intravenously for life-threatening dysrhythmias:

- For *refractory ventricular fibrillation:* **5 mg/kg** as a **bolus IV** followed by electric defibrillation. If ventricular fibrillation persists, the dose may be increased to 10 mg/kg and repeated at 15- to 30-minute intervals. Do not exceed a **maximum total dose of 30 mg/kg.**
- For *refractory or recurrent ventricular tachycardia:* Dilute 500 mg of bretylium tosylate in 50 ml of D5/W (to yield a concentration of 10 mg/ml), and give **10 mg/kg** by **IV infusion over 8 to 10 minutes.** Once that loading dose has been given, bretylium may be administered as a continuous drip at 1 to 2 mg/min.

Note: Bretylium may require 15 to 30 minutes before taking full effect.

**Incompatibility**

- May interact with **antihypertensive** medications to cause hypotension.
- May interact with **sympathomimetic** agents to potentiate their pressor effects.

# Calcium Preparations

**Therapeutic Effects**

- Reverses overdose with magnesium sulfate or calcium channel blockers (such as verapamil).
- Relieves some types of muscle spasm.
- Increases the strength of myocardial contractions.

**Indications**

- To oppose the actions of potassium in **hyperkalemia.**
- As an **antidote to magnesium sulfate.**
- As an **antidote to verapamil** overdose.
- To relieve muscle spasm and pain from **bites** of **black widow spider, scorpion,** and **Portuguese man-of-war.**

**Contraindications**

Should be used with extreme *caution* and in reduced dosage in patients taking **digitalis** preparations (e.g., digoxin).

**Side Effects**

- When given to a patient who has been taking digitalis or when given too rapidly, calcium can cause **sudden death** from ventricular fibrillation.
- Rapid IV administration may cause a metallic or chalky taste, **paresthesias,** vasodilation, **hypotension,** and a feeling that a **"wave of heat"** is passing through the body.

**How Supplied**

**Calcium chloride:** 10 ml of a 10% solution in prefilled syringes (= 13.6 mEq $Ca^{++}$)
**Calcium gluconate:** 10 ml of a 10% solution in prefilled syringes (= 4.8 mEq $Ca^{++}$)

**Administration and Dosage**

Calcium preparations are given as a **slow intravenous injection.**

For *magnesium sulfate overdose, verapamil toxicity,* or severe muscle pain after *black widow spider bite:* Calcium gluconate, **10 ml of a 10% solution IV.**

## Calcium Preparations (continued)

**Incompatibility**

Should not be given in the same infusion with **sodium bicarbonate,** since calcium chloride will combine with sodium bicarbonate to form an insoluble precipitate (calcium carbonate, i.e., chalk).

# Corticosteroids

Solu-Cortef (hydrocortisone)
Solu-Medrol (methylprednisolone)
Decadron, Dexacort (dexamethasone)

**Therapeutic Effects**

Not fully understood. May diminish the severity of allergic and inflammatory reactions.

**Indications**

- As an ancillary measure in the treatment of **severe allergic states,** such as anaphylaxis or status asthmaticus.
- For treatment and perhaps prevention of **acute mountain sickness.**
- May prove useful in minimizing damage from **spinal cord injury.**
- To treat certain **pulmonary injuries,** such as near drowning, aspiration, and toxic inhalations. (*Note:* This use of corticosteroids is controversial.)

**Contraindications**

No contraindications to a single IV dose in the field.

**Side Effects**

If administered too rapidly, especially in large doses, may cause **hypotension** and **cardiovascular collapse.** Otherwise there are no significant side effects to a *single dose* of corticosteroid. (Long-term administration of corticosteroids is associated with many side effects.)

**How Supplied**

- *Hydrocortisone:* Powder in vials of 100 mg, 250 mg, 500 mg, and 1,000 mg, for reconstitution in the diluent fluid supplied.
- *Methylprednisolone:* Powder in vials containing 40 mg, 125 mg, 500 mg, and 1,000 mg, for reconstitution in the diluent fluid supplied.
- *Dexamethasone:* 1-ml, 5-ml, and 25-ml vials; in 1-ml prefilled syringes, each containing 4 mg/ml.

# Corticosteroids (continued)

**Administration and Dosage**

- For *severe allergic reactions:*
  Hydrocortisone: **100 mg** slowly IV.
  Methylprednisolone: **20 mg** slowly IV.
  Dexamethasone: **4 mg** slowly IV.
- For *cerebral edema* or *pulmonary injury:*
  Methylprednisolone: **50 mg** slowly IV.
  Dexamethasone: **10 mg** slowly IV.
- For *spinal cord injury:*
  Methylprednisolone: Bolus of **30 mg/kg slowly IV** followed by **5.4 mg/kg/hr** by infusion (still experimental).

**Incompatibility**

None of signficance.

# 50% Dextrose (D50)

**Therapeutic Effects**

- Rapidly restores blood sugar level to normal in states of hypoglycemia.
- Acts transiently as an osmotic diuretic.

**Indications**

- To treat suspected **hypoglycemia.**
- To treat **coma of unknown cause,** when there are no contraindications.
- In **status epilepticus** of uncertain cause.

**Contraindications**

- Intracranial hemorrhage.
- Known **stroke.**

**Side Effects**

- May precipitate severe neurologic symptoms of **Wernicke's encephalopathy** in alcoholics. For that reason, administration of D50 should be preceded by *thiamine* administration (see dosage below), which will prevent the neurologic syndrome from emerging.
- Will cause **tissue necrosis** if it infiltrates; should therefore be given only through a *rapidly flowing IV line in a large vein.*

**How Supplied**

Prefilled syringes and vials containing 50 ml of 50% dextrose (= 25 gm of dextrose).

**Administration and Dosage**

Given **intravenously through a free-flowing line,** preferably in a large vein. If possible, draw blood for serum glucose determination before administering the dextrose and confirm hypoglycemia by Dextrostix. First give **thiamine, 50 mg IV plus 50 mg IM.**

*Dosage* of dextrose: 50 ml of 50% solution (**25 gm**) slowly IV.

**Incompatibility**

None of significance.

# Diazepam

Valium

**Therapeutic Effects**

- Suppresses seizure activity in the motor cortex of the brain.
- Generalized central nervous system depressant.
- Muscle relaxant.

**Indications**

- To treat **status epilepticus.**
- To provide sedation prior to **cardioversion.**
- In selected cases, to relieve **overwhelming anxiety.**

**Contraindications**

- Should not be given during **pregnancy** because of possible toxic effects on the fetus.
- Should not be given to patients who have taken **alcohol** or other **sedative drugs.**
- Should not be given to patients with **respiratory depression** from any source.
- Should not be given to patients with **hypotension.**

**Side Effects**

- Possible **hypotension.**
- Depression of the **level of consciousness.**
- In the elderly, the very illl, and patients with pulmonary disease, may cause **respiratory arrest** and/or **cardiac arrest.**

**How Supplied**

Prefilled syringes, 2-ml ampules, and 10-ml vials, in a concentration of either 5 mg/ml or 10 mg/ml.

## **Diazepam** (continued)

**Administration and Dosage**

- For *status epilepticus:* Given intravenously in slow, titrated doses. Before administering the drug, check and record the patient's vital signs. Then give **2.5 mg** (0.5 ml of a 5 mg/ml concentration) **slowly IV.** Wait a few minutes, and recheck the blood pressure (BP); if it has fallen, do *not* give any more of the drug. If the BP is stable and the patient is still seizing, give another 2.5 mg slowly IV. Recheck the BP. Continue until the seizures have stopped or the BP drops, but **do not exceed a total dose of 10 mg** in the field. (In children, diazepam may be given *rectally* for status epilepticus, in a dosage of 0.5 mg/kg.)
- For *severe anxiety* that must for some reason be treated in the field: **2 to 5 mg IM.**
- For *premedication prior to cardioversion:* **5 to 10 mg slowly IV.**

**Incompatibility**

Should not be mixed with any other drugs because of possible precipitation.

# Diphenhydramine

Benadryl

**Therapeutic Effects**
- Blocks histamine effects.
- Reverses some untoward effects of phenothiazine tranquilizers.
- Inhibits motion sickness (antiemetic).
- Mild sedative.

**Indications**
- As an *adjunct to epinephrine* in the treatment of **anaphylactic shock** and **severe allergic reactions.**
- To treat **acute dystonic reactions** caused by phenothiazines like thorazine (Compazine).

**Contraindications**
- **Asthma** or **chronic obstructive pulmonary disease.**
- **Prostatic enlargement.**
- Narrow-angle (acute) **glaucoma.**
- Ulcer disease with symptoms of obstruction (vomiting).
- **Pregnancy.**
- **Nursing mothers.**

**Side Effects**

Resemble those of atropine:

- **Drowsiness,** confusion.
- **Blurring** of vision.
- **Difficulty in urination** (especially in older men).
- **Dry mouth.**
- **Wheezing;** thickened bronchial secretions.
- Headache.
- Palpitations.

**How Supplied**
- Vials of 10 or 30 ml containing 10 mg/ml.
- Vials of 10 ml containing 50 mg/ml.
- Ampules of 1 ml containing 50 mg/ml.
- Prefilled syringes containing 50 mg in 1 ml.

Note: *Check the label carefully!*

# **Diphenhydramine** (continued)

**Administration and Dosage**
For most purposes, diphenhydramine can be given by **deep intramuscular injection.**

*Dosage:* **10 to 50 mg.**

**Incompatibility**
None of significance.

# Dobutamine

Dobutrex

**Therapeutic Effects**

Primarily **beta-1 sympathomimetic** drug with some **beta-2** activity. Dobutamine increases the force of cardiac contractions (positive inotropic effect) without causing a major increase in heart rate (i.e., without a major chronotropic effect).

**Indications**

Short-term treatment of **congestive heart failure.**

**Contraindications**

- Should not be used as a first-line treatment in **hypovolemic shock,** for which fluid replacement should be given initially.
- Patients with idiopathic hypertrophic subaortic stenosis.

**Side Effects**

- **Hypertension** in 7.5% of patients; more rarely, ***hypo*****tension** (usually promptly reversed by decreasing the dosage).
- **Tachycardia.**
- May precipitate or worsen **PVCs** (premature ventricular contractions).
- **Phlebitis** at the site of the infusion.
- Rarely, nausea, headache, angina, palpitations, dyspnea.

**How Supplied**

White powder in 20-ml vials of 250 mg. (Reconstitute with 10–20 ml of normal saline or sterile water for injection.)

# Dobutamine (continued)

**Administration and Dosage**

Given as a **titrated intravenous infusion.**

To prepare the infusion, add 250 mg of dobutamine to 500 ml of D5/W, yielding a concentration of 500 μg/ml. *Start* the infusion at a rate of **2.5 μg/kg/min.** Titrate slowly upward, to a maximum dosage of 10 μg/kg/min until there is an improvement in the patient's level of consciousness or until the systolic blood pressure reaches 90 mm Hg.

**Incompatibility**

- Do not add to **sodium bicarbonate** or any other strongly alkaline solutions.
- Do not mix with any other drugs in the same intravenous bag.
- Do not use with other agents containing **sodium bisulfite** or **ethanol.**

# Dopamine

Intropin, Revimine

**Therapeutic Effects**

**Beta sympathomimetic** drug—hence causes an increase in the rate and force of cardiac contractions as well as dilatation of mesenteric and renal arteries. The latter effect promotes urine flow, and for that reason, dopamine is sometimes preferred over norepinephrine (which constricts renal arteries) in shock. Dopamine causes less increase in myocardial oxygen consumption than does isoproterenol. At low doses of dopamine ($< 10$ μg/kg/min), its beta effects predominate; at higher doses, dopamine has alpha effects as well and thus causes vasoconstriction.

**Indications**

- In resuscitation, to treat **hypotension** that comes with bradycardia or with the return of spontaneous circulation.
- To increase cardiac output in **cardiogenic shock** while maintaining good renal perfusion.

**Contraindications**

- Should not be used as a first-line therapy in **hypotension caused by hypovolemia** (e.g., hemorrhagic shock), where volume replacement should precede the use of vasopressors.
- **Pheochromocytoma** (a tumor that produces epinephrine and/or related substances).
- Should not be given in the presence of uncorrected **tachyarrhythmias** or **ventricular fibrillation.**

**Side Effects**

- Ectopic beats, tachycardia, **palpitations.**
- Nausea, vomiting.
- **Angina.**
- Headache.
- Leakage around the vein (extravasation) may cause local **tissue necrosis.**

## Dopamine (continued)

**How Supplied**

- 5-ml ampules containing 200 mg (40 mg/ml).
- 5-ml vials containing 400 mg (80 mg/ml).

Note: *Check the label carefully!*

**Administration and Dosage**

Given by **titrated intravenous infusion** (microdrip infusion set).

*Dosage:* Transfer the contents of one ampule (200 mg) of dopamine into a 250-ml bag of D5/W to yield a concentration of 800 µg/ml. *Start* the infusion at a rate of **2 to 5 µg/kg/min** (e.g., 140–350 µg/min for a 70-kg man, or roughly 0.25 ml/min of the above dilution). *Titrate* the infusion according to the state of consciousness, blood pressure, and urine flow. If a dosage higher than 20 µg/kg/min is needed, add a norepinephrine infusion instead of increasing the dopamine dosage any further.

When blood pressure support is no longer required, dopamine should be *tapered* slowly, not discontinued abruptly.

**Incompatibility**

Do not mix with **sodium bicarbonate,** since alkaline solutions may inactivate dopamine.

# Epinephrine

Adrenalin

**Therapeutic Effects**

Beta-1 sympathetic effects:

- May **restore electric activity** in asystole.
- Increases myocardial contractility.
- Lowers the threshold for defibrillation.

Beta-2 sympathetic effects:

- Acts as a **bronchodilator.**

Alpha sympathetic effects:

- Produces **vasoconstriction,** which elevates perfusion pressure and may thus improve coronary blood flow during external chest compressions.
- Vasoconstriction also helps support the blood pressure in anaphylactic shock.

**Indications**

- In **cardiac arrest,** to restore electric activity in asystole or to enhance defibrillation potential in ventricular fibrillation; also to elevate systemic vascular resistance and thereby improve perfusion pressure during CPR.
- To treat the life-threatening symptoms of **anaphylaxis.**
- To treat acute attacks of **asthma** (second-line drug).

**Contraindications**

- Must be used with *caution* in patients with **angina, hypertension,** or **hyperthyroidism.**
- **Tachyarrhythmias**.

Note: *There are no contraindications to the use of epinephrine in cardiac arrest or anaphylactic shock.*

**Side Effects**

In the patient who is not in cardiac arrest, may cause

- Palpitations from tachycardia or ectopic beats.
- **Hypertension.**
- **Angina.**

## Epinephrine (continued)

**How Supplied**

- Prefilled syringes containing 1 mg of epinephrine in 10 ml (1:10,000 solution).
- Ampules containing 1 mg of epinephrine in 1 ml (1:1,000 solution).

**Administration and Dosage**

- In *cardiac arrest,* epinephrine is given **intravenously.** *IV dosage:* 1.0 mg (**10 ml of a 1:10,000 solution**); repeat at 3- to 5-minute intervals throughout resuscitation. After each dose by peripheral IV, **flush** the line **with 20 ml of IV fluid** to ensure delivery of the drug into the central circulation. If an IV route cannot be established quickly, the drug may be instilled in the tracheobronchial tree via *endotracheal tube.* For *endotracheal instillation,* use 2 to 2.5 times the intravenous dose (i.e., **2.0–2.5 mg**).
- For *mild anaphylactic reactions:* **0.3 to 0.5 ml of 1:1,000 solution SQ.** If the reaction is due to an injection or an insect sting, also inject 0.1 to 0.2 ml of the same solution at the injection site (but *not* on fingers, toes, ears, nose, or genitalia).
- For *severe anaphylactic reactions in a patient less than 35 years old:* Give **0.1 ml/kg of 1:10,000 solution slowly IV.** If you have neither IV nor endotracheal access, give 0.5 ml of 1:1,000 solution into the vascular plexus at the base of the tongue.
- For *asthmatic attacks:* **0.3 to 0.5 ml of a 1:1,000 solution SQ.**

**Incompatibility**

- Do not mix with **sodium bicarbonate,** since alkaline solutions may inactivate epinephrine.
- May cause severe hypertension and reflex bradycardia if given to a patient taking **beta blockers,** such as propranolol.

# Epinephrine, Racemic

Vaponefrin

**Therapeutic Effects**
Bronchodilator

**Indications**

- Upper airway problems in children, especially **croup.**
- To buy time to secure the airway in **anaphylaxis** with rapidly progressive laryngeal edema (as evidenced by stridor).

**Contraindications**

- Severe **tachyarrythmias.**
- **Epiglottitis.**

**Side Effects**

- Tachycardia, **dysrhythmias,** palpitations.
- **Angina.**
- Headache, dizziness.
- Paradoxical bronchospasm if used excessively.

**How Supplied**
30-ml bottle of 2.25% solution for nebulization.

**Administration and Dosage**
Dilute **0.5 ml in 3 ml of normal saline** and **nebulize** over 10 to 15 minutes

Note: *Do not repeat dosage.*

**Incompatibility**
May induce hypertensive crisis in patients taking tricyclic or monoamine oxidase inhibitor **antidepressant drugs.**

# Flumazenil

Mazicon, Romazicon, Anexate

**Therapeutic Effects**

Antagonizes the actions of benzodiazepines on the central nervous system by competitively blocking GABA (gamma-aminobutyric acid) receptors.

**Indications**

To treat **benzodiazepine overdose.** This class of drug includes the following:

| Generic Name | Trade Name |
|---|---|
| alprazolam | Xanax |
| chlordiazepoxide | Librium |
| clonazepam | Klonopin |
| clorazepate | Tranxene |
| diazepam | Valium |
| flurazepam | Dalmane |
| halazepam | Paxipam |
| lorazepam | Ativan |
| midazolam | Versed |
| oxazepam | Serax |
| prazepam | Centrax |
| temazepam | Restoril |
| triazolam | Halcion |

**Contraindications**

- Patients who have been given a benzodiazepine for control of a potentially life-threatening condition (e.g., status epilepticus).
- Patients showing signs of serious **cyclic antidepressant overdose** or **mixed overdoses** with unknown psychoactive drugs.
- Patients with signs of or history of **seizures.**
- Known hypersensitivity to benzodiazepines or flumazenil.
- Use with extreme caution, if at all, in patients with **head injury** (may precipitate seizures).

# Flumazenil (continued)

**Side Effects**

- **Seizures** may occur in patients who are relying on benzodiazepine effects to control convulsions or who have ingested large doses of other drugs.
- **Headache,** sweating, flushing.
- Nausea and **vomiting.**
- Dizziness, ataxia, agitation, strange feelings.
- Blurred vision.
- **Death** has occurred in patients who ingested large amounts of other drugs or who had serious underlying diseases.

**How Supplied**

5-ml multiple-dose vials containing 0.5 mg/ml.
10-ml multiple-dose vials containing 0.5 mg/ml.

**Administration and Dosage**

Give **0.2 mg** (2 ml) **by IV push over 15 to 30 seconds.** If no response occurs after 30 seconds, may give another 0.3 mg IV push, followed by 0.5 mg IV push every minute until the patient responds or a cumulative dose of 5 mg has been given (80% of patients with pure benzodiazepine overdose will respond within 3 minutes). Should be administered into a **freely running intravenous infusion in a large vein** to minimize pain at the injection site.

**Incompatibility**

Do not use in **mixed drug overdoses,** since the toxic effects (such as seizures) of other drugs taken in overdose may be unmasked by reversal of benzodiazepine effects.

# Furosemide

Lasix, Fusid

**Therapeutic Effects**

Potent **diuretic,** causing excretion of large volumes of urine within 5 to 30 minutes of administration, thus useful in ridding the body of excess fluid in conditions of fluid overload (e.g., congestive heart failure).

**Indications**

- For the treatment of fluid overload in **congestive heart failure.**
- For some cases of transfusion reaction.

**Contraindications**

- **Pregnancy.**
- **Hypovolemic states.**
- **Hypokalemia** (suspect in patients on chronic diuretic therapy with prominent P waves and flattened T waves on the electrocardiogram).

**Side Effects**

Acute side effects may include

- Nausea and **vomiting.**
- Potassium depletion, leading to cardiac **dysrhythmias.**
- **Dehydration.**
- Acute urinary retention in an uncatheterized male.

Adverse reactions are more likely in the elderly, so avoid giving furosemide to elderly patients in the prehospital phase.

**How Supplied**

- Prefilled syringes of 2 ml, 4 ml, and 10 ml containing 10 mg/ml.
- Ampules of 2 ml, 4 ml, and 10 ml containing 10 mg/ml.

## Furosemide (continued)

**Administration and Dosage**

In the field, furosemide is given **intravenously.** If transport time will be more than 15 minutes, the patient should have a urinary catheter.

*Dosage:* **20 to 40 mg slowly IV** (injected over 1–2 minutes).

**Incompatibility**

Should not be given to patients taking **lithium** (furosemide may block the renal excretion of lithium and thereby cause lithium to accumulate in the body to toxic levels).

# Ipecac, Syrup of

**Therapeutic Effects**

**Induces vomiting** and thereby effectively empties the stomach of ingested poisons or drugs taken in excess.

**Indications**

To induce vomiting in **poisoning** or **drug overdose** by ingestion in a conscious patient.

**Contraindications**

- **Stupor** or **coma.**
- **Absent gag reflex.**
- **Seizures.**
- **Pregnancy.**
- Acute **myocardial infarction.**
- Children **under 6 months old.**
- Ingestion of
  1. **Corrosives** (strong acids or alkalis).
  2. Volatile **hydrocarbons.**
  3. **Strychnine** or **iodides.**

**Side Effects**

None from the syrup of ipecac itself, *but* the patient induced to vomit—by whatever means—is at risk of aspiration.

**How Supplied**

16-oz (480-ml) bottles containing 70 mg/ml.

**Administration and Dosage**

Syrup of ipecac is given **by mouth.**

*Dosage:*

- Children: **3 to 5 teaspoons** (15–25 ml) followed by a glass of water.
- Adults: **1 to 2 tablespoons** (30–60 ml) followed by a glass of water.

The patient should be encouraged to walk around after taking the syrup of ipecac, until he feels the urge to vomit. He should then be positioned with his head lower than his waist and his face over a suitable receptacle. Save a sample of the emesis for laboratory analysis. Follow with activated charcoal.

**Incompatibility**

None.

# Isoetharine

Bronkosol

**Therapeutic Effects**

**Sympathomimetic** drug with predominant **beta-2** activity; therefore relaxes bronchial smooth muscle to produce **bronchodilation.**

**Indications**

For control of bronchospasm in **asthma** and other conditions complicated by bronchospasm, such as **chronic obstructive pulmonary disease.**

**Contraindications**

- **Allergy** to any components of the mixture, including the acetone sodium bisulfite, to which some asthmatics are sensitive.
- Must be used with *caution* in patients with **angina, hypertension,** and **tachyarrhythmias.**

**Side Effects**

- **Tachycardia,** palpitations.
- Headache, **dizziness,** weakness.
- **Anxiety,** restlessness.
- May cause **paradoxical bronchospasm** after excessive use.
- May make **sputum pink** (which can be mistaken for hemoptysis).

**How Supplied**

- In metered-dose inhalers (MDI).
- As a 1% solution in bottles of 10 ml and 30 ml.

**Administration and Dosage**

Given by **metered-dose inhaler** *or* by **nebulizer.**

*Dosage for MDI:* **1 to 2 inhalations,** preferably with a spacer.

*Dosage for nebulizer:* Dilute **0.5 ml in 3 ml of saline,** and administer **over 15 to 20 minutes.**

**Incompatibility**

**Do not administer with epinephrine** or other sympathomimetic agents, since together they may cause excessive tachycardia.

# Isoproterenol

Isuprel

**Therapeutic Effects**

Pure **beta sympathomimetic** agent, hence increases the rate, force, and automaticity of the heart and decreases peripheral resistance (through vasodilatation). In addition, relaxes bronchial smooth muscles to produce bronchodilation.

**Indications**

No longer a first-line drug for any indication.

In the field, used as a *last resort* in **symptomatic bradycardia** when atropine and epinephrine have not been effective. Also used (rarely) to treat inadvertent overdose with beta blockers such as labetalol.

**Contraindications**

- Since isoproterenol markedly increases myocardial oxygen demand, the drug should not be given in **acute myocardial infarction** or **cardiogenic shock.**
- Should not be given when there are **tachyarrhythmias.**
- Should not be given together with **epinephrine,** since the effects may be additive.

**Side Effects**

- **Tachycardia,** palpitations, **angina,** and sometimes **PVCs** (premature ventricular contractions).
- May increase infarct size in acute myocardial infarction.
- Flushing, sweating, **hypotension.**
- **Anxiety,** dizziness, tremor.

**How Supplied**

Solution of 0.2 mg/ml in ampules of 1 ml and 5 ml.

# Isoproterenol (continued)

**Administration and Dosage**
Given by **titrated intravenous infusion** (microdrip administration set). To prepare the infusion, add 1 mg (5 ml) of isoproterenol to 500 ml of D5/W to yield a solution containing 2 μg/ml. *Start* the infusion at 2 μg/min (1 ml/min of the above dilution), and slowly increase the rate up to a maximum of 10 μg/min, as needed to produce an increase in heart rate to 60 beats/min.

**Incompatibility**
Do not mix with **sodium bicarbonate,** since isoproterenol may be inactivated by alkaline solutions.

# Labetalol

Normodyne, Trandate

**Therapeutic Effects**

- **Alpha** sympathetic **blocker** that reverses vasoconstriction.
- Also a **beta blocker,** opposing the effects of beta agents on the heart, blood vessels, and lungs.

Thus labetalol can lower blood pressure (vasodilator effect) without producing the reflex tachycardia that usually accompanies a fall in blood pressure. The net effect, then, is to **reduce heart rate, cardiac output, and peripheral resistance.**

**Indications**

Control of blood pressure in **hypertensive crisis.**

**Contraindications**

- **Asthma.**
- **Cardiac failure.**
- **Heart block.**
- **Cardiogenic shock.**
- **Severe bradycardia.**

**Side Effects**

- **Postural hypotension** if the patient is allowed to assume an upright posture within 3 hours of receiving the drug.
- Occasional **dizziness** and **nausea.**

**How Supplied**

20-ml and 40-ml ampules and 20-ml and 60-ml multidose vials in a concentration of 5 mg/ml.

# Labetalol (continued)

**Administration and Dosage**
Best given by **continuous IV infusion:** Add the contents of two 20-ml ampules (200 mg) to 160 ml of D5/W to yield a concentration of 1 mg/ml. Administer at a rate of **2 mg/min** (2 ml/min).

- *The patient must remain supine throughout the administration of the drug and for at least 3 hours afterward.*
- *Monitor* blood pressure, pulse, and electrocardiogram throughout.
- Have atropine and isoproterenol ready.

**Incompatibility**
None of significance.

# Lidocaine

Xylocaine

**Therapeutic Effects**

- Suppresses ventricular ectopic activity by decreasing the excitability of heart muscle and of the electric conduction system of the heart.
- Local anesthesia.

**Indications**

Lidocaine is the drug of first choice:

- To **suppress premature ventricular contractions** (PVCs) when
  1. They occur in the context of *myocardial ischemia.*
  2. They are *frequent* (more than 6/min).
  3. They occur in *salvos* (two or more in a row).
  4. They fall on the T wave (*R-on-T* phenomenon).
  5. They are *multifocal* (having different shapes and sizes).
- To treat **ventricular tachycardia.**
- To treat **wide-complex PSVT** (paroxysmal supraventricular tachycardia) of uncertain type.

*Note:* Lidocaine is no longer considered useful as a prophylactic measure against ventricular fibrillation in acute myocardial infarction.

**Contraindications**

- Known history of **allergy** to lidocaine or local anesthetics (e.g., Novocain).
- Second- or third-degree **heart block.**
- PVCs occurring in the context of **sinus bradycardia** or sinus arrest.
- **Idioventricular rhythm.**

# Lidocaine (continued)

**Side Effects**

- By decreasing the force of cardiac contractions as well as decreasing peripheral resistance, may cause a **fall in cardiac output and blood pressure.**
- May cause **numbness, drowsiness,** or **confusion.**
- Anxiety, **tremors,** muscle twitching, slurred speech, paresthesias.
- When given in high doses, especially to the elderly or to patients in heart failure, may cause **seizures.**

**How Supplied**

- Ampules and prefilled syringes containing 100 mg in 5 ml (20 mg/ml) for bolus injection.
- Vials of 1 or 2 gm for making up an infusion solution.

**Administration and Dosage**

Given by **intravenous bolus and infusion.** If an intravenous route cannot be established, lidocaine may be given via the **endotracheal tube.**

*Dosage:*

- *In cardiac arrest, for recurrent VF (ventricular fibrillation):* **1.5 mg/kg IV bolus.** May be repeated in 5 to 10 minutes if needed. When spontaneous circulation returns, start an **infusion of 2 mg/min.** To prepare the infusion, add 0.5 gm (500 mg) of lidocaine to 250 ml of D5/W, yielding a solution of 2 mg/ml. Use a microdrip infusion set for administration.
- *For PVCs and VT (ventricular tachycardia):* Give **1 mg/kg IV push,** followed by an **infusion of 2 mg/min.** Prepare the infusion as described above.

**Incompatibility**

Do not give together with **beta blockers** or **dopamine.**

# Lorazepam

Ativan, Lorivan

**Therapeutic Effects**

- A benzodiazepine (in the same family as diazepam).
- Suppresses seizure activity in the motor cortex of the brain.
- Generalized central nervous system depressant.
- Produces short-term retrograde amnesia.

**Indications**

In prehospital care, the *treatment of choice* to control seizures in **status epilepticus.** Administered *only* to patients with active convulsions, not to those whose seizures have stopped.

**Contraindications**

- Acute narrow-angle **glaucoma.**
- **Hepatic or renal failure.**
- Known sensitivity to benzodiazepines.

**Side Effects**

- **Respiratory depression.**
- **Bradycardia, hypotension.**
- Excessive **sleepiness,** especially in patients over 50 years old.
- Rarely: confusion, delirium, hallucinations.
- Enhanced sensitivity to alcoholic beverages more than 24 hours after receiving injectable lorazepam.
- Inadvertent arterial injection may produce arteriospasm resulting in gangrene.

**How Supplied**

- Tubex Sterile Cartridge-Needle Units in concentrations of 2 mg/ml and 4 mg/ml.
- In single-dose (1 ml) and multiple-dose (10 ml) vials in concentrations of 2 mg/ml or 4 mg/ml.

## **Lorazepam** (continued)

**Administration and Dosage**

- *Adults:* **0.1 mg/kg slowly IV** (start with 2–4 mg IV push at 2 mg/min); **must be diluted** in an equal volume of diluent; may repeat dose once after 15 to 20 minutes if first dose does not control seizures.
- *Children:* **0.05 to 0.5 mg/kg** diluted in an equal volume of diluent and given very slowly IV.

In both children and adults, injection must be made *slowly* with repeated aspirations to confirm that the needle is still in the vein.

**Incompatibility**

- Should not be used with other **CNS depressants** because of additive effects.
- When used concomitantly with **scopolamine,** there is an increased incidence of hallucinations, oversedation, and irrational behavior.

# Magnesium Sulfate

**Therapeutic Effects**

- Central nervous system depressant.
- Stabilizes muscle cell membranes by interacting with the sodium/potassium exchange system.
- Smooth muscle relaxation, hence vasodilation and bronchodilation.

**Indications**

- For the treatment of **eclampsia.**
- For **prophylaxis of cardiac dysrhythmias** in acute myocardial infarction.
- For treatment of selected **tachyarrhythmias.**
- For the management of **acute asthmatic attacks.**

**Contraindications**

- **Renal disease.**
- **Heart block.**

**Side Effects**

Excessive dose may cause **respiratory depression** or even **cardiac arrest.**

**How Supplied**

Ampules of 10%, 25%, or 50% solution.

# Magnesium Sulfate (continued)

**Administration and Dosage**

In the field, given by **slow intravenous injection.** The patient should be monitored by electrocardiogram and also watched closely for respiratory depression. Deep tendon reflexes (e.g., knee jerk) should be tested frequently; if deep tendon reflexes become absent, the patient may be overdosed with magnesium, and it may be necessary to administer calcium gluconate as an antidote.

- For *eclampsia:* **2 to 4 gm IV** (i.e., 20–40 ml of a 10% solution) given **over at least 3 minutes.**
- For *acute myocardial infarction:* Add **2.4 gm** to 50 ml of D5/W, and infuse **over 20 to 60 minutes.**
- For *tachyarrhythmias:* **2 gm IV over 1 minute.**
- For *acute asthmatic attacks:* **1.2 gm in 50 ml of saline over 20 minutes.**

Keep calcium gluconate (10 ml of a 10% solution) ready in the event of inadvertent overdose and respiratory depression.

**Incompatibility**

None of significance.

# Mannitol

Osmitrol

**Therapeutic Effects**

Because it remains in the vascular space, mannitol acts as an **osmotic diuretic,** to draw fluid out of cells and promote excretion of fluid from the body.

**Indications**

- For the treatment of **cerebral edema** after closed head injury, cardiac arrest, and other conditions.
- To promote diuresis and thereby minimize the damaging effects of myoglobinuria in **crush injury** or **electric injury.**
- To promote diuresis in selected **drug overdoses.**

**Contraindications**

- **Anuria** (absence of urine flow) or severe renal impairment.
- **Intracranial hemorrhage.**
- **Pregnancy.**
- **Dehydration** or sodium depletion.

**Side Effects**

- **Headache** and **nausea** in conscious patients.
- **Fall in serum sodium** concentration.
- May precipitate **congestive heart failure** in susceptible patients.
- Extravasation will cause local **tissue necrosis.**

**How Supplied**

- As a 5% or 10% solution in 1,000 ml.
- As a 15% or 20% solution in 500 ml.

Note: *Read the label carefully!*

## Mannitol (continued)

**Administration and Dosage**

Given by **intravenous infusion** using an administration set containing an **in-line filter.**

- The solution should be inspected to be certain it does not contain crystals.
- The patient should have a **urinary catheter** in place before receiving a mannitol infusion.

*Dosage:* **500 mg/kg** by IV infusion **over 15 minutes.** (Example: For a 70-kg man, dosage is 35 gm. If you are using a 20% solution, containing 200 mg/ml, you would thus give 175 ml.)

**Incompatibility**

None of significance.

# Metaraminol

Aramine

**Therapeutic Effects**
Effects are about midway between those of epinephrine and norepinephrine; that is, metaraminol has some of the **beta sympathomimetic** properties of epinephrine (producing increasing rate and force of cardiac contractions) as well as some of the **alpha** properties of norepinephrine (producing vasoconstriction). It is used as an alternative to norepinephrine for raising the blood pressure.

**Indications**
To increase blood pressure in certain cases of **neurogenic shock** or **cardiogenic shock.**

**Contraindications**
Should not be used as first-line therapy in hypotension due to **hypovolemia,** where fliud replacement should precede the use of vasopressors.

**Side Effects**
- Essentially the same as for norepinephrine.
- Extravasation can cause local **tissue necrosis.**
- Excessive dosage leads to **sweating, headache,** and **dysrhythmias.**

**How Supplied**
1-ml ampules and 10-ml vials, in a concentration of 10 mg/ml.

**Administration and Dosage**
Given by **titrated intravenous infusion** (microdrip infusion set).

*Dosage:* To prepare the infusion, add 100 mg (10 ml) of metaraminol to 250 ml of D5/W, to yield a concentration of 0.4 mg/ml. *Start* the infusion at a rate of about **0.2 mg/min** (0.5 ml/min), and gradually increase the rate of the infusion until the systolic blood pressure reaches about 90 mm Hg.

**Incompatibility**
None of significance.

# Morphine Sulfate

**Therapeutic Effects**

- **Vasodilator:** Decreases pulmonary edema by pooling blood in the peripheral circulation ("internal phlebotomy") and thereby reducing venous return to the heart; helps as well to allay the anxiety associated with pulmonary edema.
- Potent **analgesic,** providing relief of pain in myocardial infarction and other conditions.
- Lowers myocardial oxygen consumption.

**Indications**

- To treat **pulmonary edema** associated with congestive heart failure.
- To relieve **pain** in myocardial infarction, burns, and other situations of severe pain.

**Contraindications**

- Significant **hypotension.**
- **Respiratory depression,** except that caused by pulmonary edema, where morphine may be used if ventilatory support is provided.
- **Asthma** and **chronic obstructive pulmonary disease.**
- In patients who have taken **other depressant drugs,** such as alcohol or barbiturates.
- **Head injury.**
- Possible **inferior-wall AMI** (acute myocardial infarction; relative contraindication only).
- Undiagnosed **abdominal pain.**
- Patients taking **monoamine oxidase (MAO) inhibitor** antidepressant drugs.

**Side Effects**

- **Hypotension** (most likely in volume-depleted patients).
- Increased vagal tone, leading to **bradycardia** (this effect can be reversed with atropine).
- **Respiratory depression** (this effect can be reversed with naloxone).
- **Nausea** and **vomiting.**
- **Urinary retention.**

# Morphine Sulfate (continued)

**How Supplied**

Prefilled 10-ml syringes containing 1 mg/ml.
1-ml Tubex syringe containing 10 mg/ml.

**Administration and Dosage**

Given by **titrated intravenous injections.**

*Dosage:* 0.1 mg/kg. In the field, we usually give **2 to 5 mg by slow IV push** every 5 to 30 minutes until the desired therapeutic effect is achieved. **Do not exceed 15 mg in the field.**

- If hypotension occurs, keep the patient flat, and do not give more of the drug.
- Have *atropine* and *naloxone* immediately at hand to treat possible bradycardia or respiratory depression.

**Incompatibility**

Should not be given to patients taking **tricyclic antidepressants** or **MAO inhibitors** (another type of antidepressant medication).

# Naloxone

Narcan

**Therapeutic Effects**

Specific **antidote for narcotic agents.** Reverses the effects of all narcotic drugs, including heroin, morphine, methadone, codeine, meperidine (Demerol, Pethidine), hydromorphone (Dilaudid), paregoric, fentanyl, and percodan. Also effective against pentazocine (Talwin), propoxyphene (Darvon), nalbuphine (Nubain), and butorphanol (Stadol). Naloxone will reverse stupor, coma, and respiratory depression *when they are due to narcotic overdose.* Naloxone is not usually effective in reversing coma from other causes.

**Indications**

- To treat known **narcotic overdose.**
- To treat **coma of unknown cause** when the patient has failed to respond to 50% dextrose and there is reason to suspect the possibility of narcotic overdose.

**Contraindications**

None.

**Side Effects**

- Too rapid administration may precipitate **vomiting** and **ventricular dysrhythmias.**
- Administration to people who are physically dependent on narcotics may precipitate an **acute withdrawal syndrome.** For that reason, naloxone should be given slowly, using improvement of respiratory status as an end point.
- In general, the duration of action of naloxone is shorter than that of the narcotics it is used to counteract. Thus, the patient who has been successfully roused with naloxone may **fall back into stupor or coma** as the naloxone wears off. Patients treated with naloxone must therefore be watched closely, and the dose of naloxone should be repeated as necessary.
- Naloxone has been reported to cause pulmonary edema and sudden death in very rare cases.

## Naloxone (continued)

**How Supplied**

- 1-ml ampules or prefilled syringes of 0.4 mg/ml.
- 2-ml ampules of 1 mg/ml.
- 10-ml vials of 0.4 mg/ml or 1 mg/ml.
- 1-ml and 2-ml prefilled syringes of 1 mg/ml.

Note: *Read the label carefully!*

**Administration and Dosage**

In the field, given by **slow intravenous injection,** but may be given via **endotracheal tube** (diluted) or by **intralingual injection** if intravenous access cannot be secured.

*Dosage* (for intravenous administration): Draw up **0.8 mg** of naloxone in a 10-ml syringe. Fill the remainder of the syringe with D5/W. Administer this solution *slowly IV* while monitoring the rate and depth of the patient's respirations. As soon as there is improvement in the respirations, stop giving the drug. It is preferable *not* to wake the patient up completely in the field, since many such patients "come up fighting." If there is no response to the first dose, **repeat the dose** up to two more times (i.e., **up to a total dose of 2.4 mg**). If there is still no response, suspect another cause for the patient's coma.

- For *endotracheal administration:* Dilute **0.8 mg in 5 to 10 ml of normal saline.**
- For *intralingual injection:* Give **2.0 mg** in a single injection into the vascular plexus beneath the tongue.

**Incompatibility**

None of significance.

# Nifedipine

Adalat, Procardia, Pressolat

**Therapeutic Effects**

**Calcium channel blocker,** acts by inhibiting the influx of calcium ions into cardiac and smooth muscle, thereby inhibiting the contractile process. Nifedipine thus **dilates coronary arteries, reduces afterload** (by dilating peripheral arteries), and thereby both increases myocardial blood supply *and* decreases myocardial work (thus myocardial oxygen demand).

**Indications**

- **Angina,** especially that caused by coronary artery spasm. (This is the only FDA-approved indication.)
- **Hypertensive crisis** (not yet FDA-approved for this indication).

**Contraindications**

Known **allergy** to the drug.

**Side Effects**

- May produce **excessive hypotension.**
- Dizziness.
- **Flushing** or sensations of heat.
- Weakness.
- **Nausea,** heartburn.

**How Supplied**

Soft gelatin capsule of 10 mg and 20 mg.

**Administration and Dosage**

In hypertensive crisis, use a hypodermic needle to puncture several holes in a **10-mg capsule;** then place the capsule **under the patient's tongue.** Alternatively, the patient may bite open the capsule and swallow the contents.

**Incompatibility**

May potentiate the effects of **beta blocking agents,** leading to heart failure.

# Nitroglycerin

Cardilate, Isordil, Nitrol, Sorbide, and Others

**Therapeutic Effects**

The primary pharmacologic effect of nitroglycerin and related drugs is to **relax smooth muscle,** and the effects of nitroglycerin on the cardiovascular system are chiefly due to relaxation of *vascular* smooth muscle—hence **vasodilation.**

- Nitroglycerin provides relief of pain in angina, probably by dilating coronary arteries and thereby increasing blood flow through them as well as by decreasing myocardial oxygen demand.
- Through its vasodilating action on the peripheral vessels, nitroglycerin promotes pooling of the blood in the systemic circulation ("internal phlebotomy") and decreases the resistance against which the heart has to pump (the afterload); those effects are useful in treating congestive heart failure.

**Indications**

- To relieve the pain of **angina.**
- To reduce infarct size in **AMI** (acute myocardial infarction).
- To treat selected cases of **pulmonary edema** due to congestive heart failure.
- Applied topically, to **dilate veins for venipuncture** to facilitate starting an IV.

**Contraindications**

- **Increased intracranial pressure.**
- **Glaucoma.**
- **Hypovolemia.**
- **Hypotension,** especially with brady- or tachycardia.
- **Epigastric distress or hiccups accompanying symptoms of AMI** (because they suggest *inferior-*wall AMI).

## Nitroglycerin (continued)

**Side Effects**

- Transient, throbbing **headache.** (If the headache does *not* occur, suspect that the nitroglycerin is outdated and no longer potent.)
- **Hypotension,** dizziness, weakness.
- **Flushing,** feelings of warmth.

**How Supplied**

Many forms, including tablets, sustained-release capsules, ointments, and patches. For use in the field, tablets of 0.3 or 0.4 mg are preferred. (For topical application before starting an IV, use the ointment or paste form.)

**Administration and Dosage**

Given **sublingually** (under the tongue).

*Dosage:* One **0.3- or 0.4-mg tablet under the tongue** for angina, AMI, or congestive heart failure. **May repeat once** after 3 minutes. If hypotension occurs, elevate the patient's legs and give IV fluids per the physician's order.

*For dilating a vein to facilitate starting an IV in children,* apply the nitroglycerin ointment to the skin over the vein and wait at least 5 minutes.

**Incompatibility**

Do not give to a patient who has been drinking **alcohol**.

# Nitrous Oxide

Nitronox, Entonox

**Therapeutic Effects**
Provides rapid, easily reversible relief of pain.

**Indications**
Relief of **pain** from

- Acute myocardial infarction.
- Musculoskeletal trauma.
- Burns.
- Other conditions (e.g., ureteral colic, labor).

**Contraindications**
- Any **altered state of consciousness,** such as **head injury** (nitrous oxide masks the neurologic signs one needs to monitor).
- **Chronic obstructive pulmonary disease.**
- Acute **pulmonary edema** (these patients need 100% oxygen).
- Known **pneumothorax** or **chest injury** where pneumothorax may be present (nitrous oxide collects in dead air spaces and may thus expand a pneumothorax).
- **Abdominal distention** or abdominal trauma where bowel sounds are absent.
- Major **facial injury.**
- **Shock.**
- **Decompression sickness.**
- **Air embolism** from any source.

**Side Effects**
- Light-headedness, **drowsiness.**
- Occasional nausea and **vomiting.**
- Ambulance crew may experience giddiness if the vehicle is not properly vented.

## Nitrous Oxide (continued)

**How Supplied**

In the United States, nitrous oxide for field use is supplied as Nitronox, a set containing an oxygen cylinder and a nitrous oxide cylinder, joined by a valve that regulates flow to provide a fixed 50:50 mixture of the two gases. The gas mixture is piped to the demand valve apparatus. In Canada and parts of Europe, D and E cylinders color-coded blue and white contain a premix of the two gases; such cylinders must be inverted several times before use to ensure thorough mixing.

**Administration and Dosage**

Nitrous oxide is **self-administered by inhalation.** The patient is instructed to hold the mask to his or her face, to form a tight seal around the nose and mouth, and to breathe normally. As the patient becomes drowsy, the mask will drop away from his or her face. *The patient must control the demand valve himself.* The paramedic should not hold the face mask in place for the patient, for overdosage may result.

**Incompatibility**

None of significance.

# Norepinephrine

Levophed

**Therapeutic Effects**

Chiefly an **alpha sympathomimetic** agent; therefore it increases blood pressure by constricting arteries. It also has some beta activity, although less than epinephrine, and thus increases the force of cardiac contractions.

**Indications**

- To increase blood pressure in states of low total peripheral resistance, such as **neurogenic shock** or some cases of **cardiogenic shock.**
- For **blood pressure support** after cardiopulmonary resuscitation.

**Contraindications**

- Should not be used as first-line therapy in **hypovolemic shock,** where fluid replacement should precede the use of vasopressors.
- Should not be used in patients with severe **hypoxia** or **hypercarbia.**
- Should be used with extreme *caution* in patients with **myocardial infarction,** since norepinephrine increases myocardial oxygen requirements.

## **Norepinephrine** (continued)

**Side Effects**

- **Necrosis** of tissue surrounding the IV catheter can occur if the IV infiltrates or the norepinephrine solution leaks from the vein. For that reason, the IV should be established in a large vein and checked closely before a norepinephrine drip is hung. Do *not* use hand veins or leg veins for norepinephrine infusions. If extravasation occurs, phentolamine, 5 to 10 mg in 10 to 15 ml of saline, should be infiltrated as soon as possible into the area of extravasation to prevent sloughing of soft tissues.
- Within the therapeutic range, there are few other side effects. However, if the IV is inadvertently speeded up ("runaway IV") and the patient receives more than the therapeutic dose, he may experience severe **headache, sweating, nausea, vomiting, anxiety, ventricular dysrhythmias,** and **severe hypertension.**

**How Supplied**

Ampules of 4 ml containing 4 mg (1 mg/ml).

**Administration and Dosage**

Given by **titrated intravenous infusion** (microdrip infusion set). To make up the infusion, add 4 mg (4 ml) of norepinephrine to 500 ml of D5/W to yield a solution containing 8 μg/ml. *Start* the infusion at **4 μg/min** (0.5 ml/min of the above dilution), and slowly increase the rate, rechecking the blood pressure after each increase, until the systolic blood pressure reaches about 90 mm Hg. Run the infusion at the rate necessary to maintain that level of blood pressure.

**Incompatibility**

- May cause severe, prolonged hypertension in patients taking **antidepressant medications.**
- Do not administer norepinephrine in the same IV line with **alkaline solutions** (e.g., sodium bicarbonate), which may inactivate the norepinephrine.

# Oxygen

## Therapeutic Effects

Reverses the deleterious effects of hypoxemia on the brain, heart, and other tissues.

## Indications

Any condition in which systemic or local hypoxemia may be present:

- Cardiac or **respiratory arrest** (given with artificial ventilation).
- **Dyspnea** or **respiratory distress** from any cause.
- **Chest pain.**
- **Shock.**
- **Coma** from any cause.
- **Chest trauma.**
- **Near drowning.**
- **Pulmonary edema.**
- **Toxic inhalations** (smoke, carbon monoxide, chemicals).
- Acute **asthmatic attack.**
- Acute **decompensation of COPD** (chronic obstructive pulmonary disease).
- **Stroke, head injury.**
- **Status epilepticus.**
- Any patient in **critical condition.**

## Contraindications

**None.** May depress respirations in *rare* patients with COPD. That is *not* a contraindication to the use of oxygen but simply means that such patients must be closely monitored and assisted to breathe if the respiratory rate declines.

## Side Effects

None when given for short periods (less than 24 hours) to adults.

# Oxygen (continued)

**How Supplied**

As a compressed gas in cylinders of various sizes.

To calculate **how long the oxygen in a cylinder will last:**

$$\text{Duration of flow} = \frac{(\text{gauge pressure} - 200\ \text{psi}) \times C}{\text{flow rate (L/min)}}$$

where C = the cylinder constant.

*Cylinder Constants*

D cylinder = 0.16 L/psi
E cylinder = 0.26 L/psi
G cylinder = 2.41 L/psi
M cylinder = 1.56 L/psi

**Administration and Dosage**

Administered by **inhalation** from a mask, nasal cannula, endotracheal tube, etc. (see table). A patent airway and adequate ventilation must be ensured. Dosage depends on the condition being treated. For cardiac arrest and other conditions of large shunt, **100% oxygen** should be given as soon as possible.

**Incompatibility**

Oxygen supports combustion, so it should not be given where there is **open flame,** where people are smoking, and so forth.

## *Oxygen Delivery Systems*

| Device | Flow Rate Used (L/min) | % $O_2$ Delivered | Comments |
|---|---|---|---|
| Nasal catheter | 6–8 | 30–50 | Do not use in comatose patient. |
| **Nasal cannula** | 4–6 | 25–40 | Usually well tolerated. **Device of choice** when very high oxygen concentrations are not needed. |
| Venturi masks<br>24%<br>28%<br>35%<br>40% | <br>4<br>4<br>8<br>8 | <br>24<br>28<br>35<br>40 | Useful in long-term treatment of patients with COPD. Limited value in the field. |
| Partial rebreathing mask | 6–12 | 35–60 | |
| **Nonrebreathing mask** | 10–12 | 90 | **Device of choice** for administering high oxygen concentration to a patient who is breathing. |
| **Pocket mask** | 10–12 | 90 | **Preferred** device for artificial ventilation of a nonbreathing patient. |

**_Oxygen Delivery Systems_** (continued)

| Device | Flow Rate Used (L/min) | % $O_2$ Delivered | Comments |
|---|---|---|---|
| Bag-valve-mask | 10–12 | 40–60 | For artificial ventilation. |
| Bag-valve-mask with oxygen reservoir | 10–12 | 90 | For artificial ventilation. |
| Demand valve-mask | 50–150 | 100 | Useful principally in pulmonary edema. Contraindicated in children. |

# Oxytocin

Pitocin, Syntocinon

**Therapeutic Effects**

Promotes contraction of the uterus toward its normal size after delivery; the contracting uterine muscle squeezes down on uterine blood vessels and thereby reduces postpartum bleeding.

**Indications**

To improve uterine contraction and thereby **control postpartum bleeding** *after delivery of the placenta.*

**Contraindications**

- Previous **cesarean section.**
- **Twin pregnancy**, before the birth of the second baby.

**Side Effects**

Side effects are rare when oxytocin is given after the second stage of labor but may include

- **Nausea** and **vomiting.**
- Cardiac **dysrhythmias.**
- Allergic **reactions** to the drug.

**How Supplied**

Ampules and prefilled syringes containing 10 units in 1 ml.

**Administration and Dosage**

Given by **intravenous infusion.** Inject **10 units** (1 ml) of oxytocin into **1,000 ml of normal saline**, and infuse at the rate ordered by the physician.

**Incompatibility**

Do not administer to patients receiving **vasopressor drugs,** as the combination may cause dangerous levels of hypertension.

# Pralidoxime (2-PAM)

Protopam

**Therapeutic Effects**

Reactivates cholinesterase (mainly outside the CNS) that has been inactivated by organophosphate pesticides or related poisons, thereby allowing the neuromuscular junction to function normally again. Its main action is to relieve paralysis of the muscles of respiration. Less effective in relieving respiratory center paralysis, for which atropine is required.

**Indications**

For **severe organophosphate poisoning.**

**Contraindications**

There are no absolute contraindications in a life-threatening emergency.

**Side Effects**

- Mild to moderate **pain** at the site of injection 40 to 60 minutes after administration.
- Blurred vision, double vision.
- Dizziness, headache, drowsiness.
- When used with atropine, the **effects of atropinization** (flushing, tachycardia, dry mouth) may **occur earlier** than when atropine is used alone.

**How Supplied**

20-ml vials of 1 gm of white to off-white porous cake. (Solution is prepared by adding 20 ml of sterile water for injection.)

## Pralidoxime (2-PAM) (continued)

**Administration and Dosage**
Given as an **intravenous infusion:**

- Most effective if administered immediately after poisoning; unlikely to be helpful if more than 36 hours have elapsed since the poisoning.
- Do not administer until the patient has been fully atropinized.

*Dosage:*

- *Adults:* **1 to 2 gm in 100 ml of saline over 15 to 30 minutes.** After about an hour, a second dose of 1 to 2 gm may be indicated.
- *Children:* **20 to 40 mg/kg IV over 15 to 30 minutes.**

**Incompatibility**
Do not give **morphine, theophylline, aminophylline,** or **succinylcholine** to patients with organophosphate poisoning.

# Propranolol

Inderal, Deralin

**Therapeutic Effects**

Nonselective **beta-1 and beta-2 blocker**; thus it opposes the effects of beta agents on the heart, lungs, and blood vessels. The most important effects are on the heart, where propranolol

- Decreases the sinus rate.
- Slows atrial conduction.
- Delays conduction though the AV (atrioventricular) node.
- Depresses spontaneous electric activity and muscular force.

**Indications**

- Control of **supraventricular tachycardias.**
- Prevention of recurrent **ventricular tachycardia.**
- To slow the ventricular rate in **atrial flutter** and **atrial fibrillation** when digitalis is contraindicated.
- To reduce the incidence of ventricular fibrillation **after acute myocardial infarction** in patients who did not receive thrombolytic therapy.

**Contraindications**

- **Asthma** or **chronic obstructive pulmonary disease.**
- Patients with **hay fever** during the pollen season.
- Sinus bradycardia; second- or third-degree **heart block.**
- Congestive **heart failure.**
- Any state in which **cardiac function** is **depressed** (e.g., immediately after resuscitation from cardiac arrest).

**Side Effects**

- **Hypotension** and/or **heart failure.**
- **Bronchospasm.**
- **Nausea** and **vomiting.**
- May **mask symptoms of hypoglycemia** in diabetics.

# **Propranolol** (continued)

**How Supplied**

Ampules of 1 ml containing 1 mg.

**Administration and Dosage**

In the field, given by **slow intravenous injection.**

*Dosage:* **1 mg** injected IV **over 5 minutes.** If there is no response, a second dose of 0.5 mg may be given slowly IV 5 to 10 minutes after the first dose.

**Incompatibility**

Do not give together with **sympathomimetics** (such as epinephrine), **aminophylline**, or known cardiac depressants.

# Sodium Bicarbonate

**Therapeutic Effects**

A **buffer.** By neutralizing excess acid, helps return the blood and body fluids toward a physiologic pH, in which metabolic processes and sympathomimetic agents work more effectively.

**Indications**

- To treat **metabolic acidosis,** as in
  1. Certain **poisonings** (e.g., ethylene glycol).
  2. **Shock** and other low-output states (e.g., after resuscitation from cardiac arrest).
- To treat **hyperkalemia** (high serum potassium).
- To promote the excretion of some types of **barbiturate** taken in **overdose.**
- To promote excretion of myoglobin in **crush injuries** and **electrocution.**
- In some cases of **status asthmaticus.**
- In **prolonged CPR.**

**Contraindications**

- **Hypokalemia** (low serum potassium), sometimes detectable by large, prominent P waves, large U waves, and flattened T waves on the ECG.
- Conditions in which the patient cannot tolerate a salt load, such as **congestive heart failure.**

**Side Effects**

- Because each milliequivalent of bicarbonate comes along with a milliequivalent of sodium, sodium bicarbonate has the same effect as any other salt-containing solution; that is, it **increases the vascular volume**. Three 50-ml syringes of sodium bicarbonate (1 mEq/ml) contain approximately the same amount of salt as 1 liter of normal saline. Patients in borderline heart failure cannot tolerate salt loads of that magnitude and may be plunged into **pulmonary edema.**

## Sodium Bicarbonate (continued)

- Administration of sodium bicarbonate **lowers the serum potassium**. When bicarbonate is used to treat hyperkalemia, that is the desired effect. However, in cardiac patients, the heart becomes irritable if the potassium falls too low, and **dysrhythmias** may occur, especially in patients taking diuretics.
- Sodium bicarbonate administration transiently **raises the arterial $PCO_2$,** so its administration must be accompanied by controlled hyperventilation (e.g., with a bag-valve-mask) to blow off the excess carbon dioxide.

**How Supplied**
Vials and prefilled syringes of 50 ml containing 1 mEq/ml.

**Administration and Dosage**
Given by **bolus injection.**

*Dosage:*

- For *cardiac arrest*: If used at all, **1 mEq/kg** after the first 10 minutes of CPR. Acidosis should thereafter be prevented by hyperventilating the patient.
- For *other conditions*: As ordered by the physician.

**Incompatibility**

- Do not give together with **calcium salts,** for the combination will produce a chalky precipitate of calcium carbonate.
- Do not give together with **sympathomimetic drugs** (e.g., epinephrine), which will be inactivated in an alkaline solution.

# Streptokinase

Streptase, Varidase, Kabikinase

**Therapeutic Effects**

**Lyses** (dissolves) **thrombi** that have recently formed in the coronary arteries, thereby enabling renewed blood flow through blocked coronaries in the acute phase of myocardial infarction.

**Indications**

Evolving **acute myocardial infarction** within the first 6 hours if inclusion criteria are met (see table).

**Contraindications**

- Active **internal bleeding** (e.g., peptic ulcer).
- Recent **stroke** or **intracranial surgery.**
- Severe, uncontrolled **hypertension.**
- Recent **trauma, surgery.**
- Patient taking **oral anticoagulant medications.**
- Insulin-dependent **diabetes mellitus.**

**Side Effects**

- **Bleeding** tendency; fatal hemorrhage has occurred.
- **Allergic reactions** to the drug, with itching, hives, flushing, nausea, headache, and myalgias (can be minimized by pretreatment with diphenhydramine).
- **Fever.**
- **Hypotension.**
- Reperfusion **dysrhythmias.**

**How Supplied**

6.5-ml vials of powdered drug with a color-coded label corresponding to the amount of purified streptokinase in each vial:

- Green: 250,000 IU.
- Blue: 750,000 IU.
- Red: 1,500,000 IU.

## Streptokinase (continued)

**Administration and Dosage**
Given by **intravenous infusion,** using an **in-line filter** to screen out particulate matter.
Reconstitute the powdered drug with 5 ml of normal saline injected down the side of the vial. Then roll the vial gently (don't shake it) to dissolve the powder. Inspect for particulate matter.

*Dosage:* **1,500,000 IU** diluted in at least 45 ml of normal saline and **infused over 60 minutes.**

**Incompatibility**
None of significance.

### *Criteria for Thrombolytic Therapy*

| Inclusion criteria | Exclusion criteria |
|---|---|
| Alert and able to give informed consent | Significant bleeding or known bleeding disorder |
| Age > 30 years | Stroke or transient ischemic attack |
| Chest pain for > 20 minutes and < 6 hours | History of gastrointestinal or genitourinary bleeding |
| Pain not relieved by sublingual nitroglycerin | Patient taking oral anticoagulant medication |
| Systolic BP > 80 and < 180 mm Hg | Insulin-dependent diabetes mellitus |
| Diastolic BP < 120 mm Hg | Terminal illness |
| Systolic pressure difference between the two arms < 20 mm Hg | Severe hypertension (systolic BP > 180 mm Hg, diastolic BP > 120 mm Hg) |
| ECG: S–T elevation of > 1 mm in two adjacent leads | Intravenous cannulas at noncompressible sites |

# Succinylcholine

Anectine

**Therapeutic Effects**

Short-acting skeletal muscle relaxant that works by depolarizing the receptors on skeletal muscle. By occupying those receptors, it prevents the normal transmitting chemical from reaching the receptors and thereby **blocks neuromuscular transmission.** The result is a transient paralysis of skeletal muscles.

**Indications**

To facilitate **endotracheal intubation.**

**Contraindications**

- Patients known to have had **problems during anesthesia** in the past.
- Penetrating **eye injury.**
- Severe **burns.**
- **Organophosphate poisoning.**
- Known **neuromuscular disease** (e.g., myasthenia gravis).
- Operator who is **not highly skilled in intubation.**
- Patients in whom you **cannot control the airway manually.**

**Side Effects**

- Produces generalized **muscle fasciculations** immediately after administration (depolarizing effect).
- **Hypersalivation** (may be prevented by pretreating with atropine).
- **Bronchospasm.**
- **Bradycardia** (may be prevented by pretreating with atropine).
- Prolonged **respiratory depression.**
- In very rare cases, **malignant hyperpyrexia,** heralded by muscle rigidity, tachycardia, hypertension.

**How Supplied**

20-ml vials containing 20 mg/ml.
2-ml and 5-ml ampules of 20 mg/ml.
Should be stored in refrigerator.

## Succinylcholine (continued)

**Administration and Dosage**

Given by **intravenous bolus injection.**

1. Preoxygenate the patient for at least 3 minutes with 100% oxygen.
2. Have all **intubation equipment ready.**
3. Have **atropine, 0.01 mg/kg** drawn up in a syringe and ready to administer. Give for bradycardia or hypersecretion.
4. Premedicate:
   - Awake adults: 3–5 mg of *diazepam* slowly IV.
   - Patients with head injury: *Lidocaine,* 1 mg/kg IV.
   - Children: *Atropine,* 0.01 mg/kg IV.
5. Give succinylcholine, **1 mg/kg IV.**
6. Wait until fasciculations have stopped.
7. Have an assistant apply **cricoid pressure** to block the esophagus.
8. **Intubate** the trachea.
9. Provide **controlled ventilation** with 100% oxygen until the patient resumes breathing spontaneously (usually within 4–6 minutes, but may take longer).

**Incompatibility**

Drugs that may add to the paralytic effects of succinylcholine should not be given: **oxytocin, procainamide, lidocaine, magnesium salts, beta blockers** (e.g., propranolol).

# Terbutaline

Bricanyl, Brethine, Brethaire, Bricalin

**Therapeutic Effects**

Beta sympathomimetic agent affecting primarily the bronchial musculature rather than the myocardium (i.e., a **beta-2** agent). Terbutaline thus relaxes bronchial smooth muscle and thereby **relieves bronchospasm** in asthma.

**Indications**

- Moderate to severe **asthma.**
- Reversible bronchospasm in **chronic obstructive pulmonary disease.**

**Contraindications**

- Should be used with *caution* in patients with **angina, hypertension,** or **cardiac dysrhythmias.**
- Manufacturer does not recommend use in **children less than 12 years old.**

**Side Effects**

- **Tremor** and nervousness.
- **Palpitations,** dizziness.
- Sometimes transient **headache, sweating, drowsiness, nausea,** and **muscle cramps.**

**How Supplied**

Several forms, but for field use, as an alternative to subcutaneous epinephrine, the solution for subcutaneous injection is preferred. That solution is supplied as 1-ml ampules containing 1 mg of terbutaline (1 mg/ml).

**Administration and Dosage**

In the field, given primarily by **subcutaneous injection.**

*Dosage:*

- Children: **0.01 mg/kg SQ**; may repeat in 15 minutes.
- Adults: **0.25 mg** (0.25 ml) **SQ** over the lateral deltoid.

May also be given by **nebulizer** in a dosage of **0.03 mg/kg** added to 3 ml of normal saline.

**Incompatibility**

Do not give together with other **sympathomimetic drugs** (e.g., epinephrine).

# Thiamine (Vitamin $B_1$)

**Therapeutic Effects**

Acts as a coenzyme in carbohydrate metabolism and is therefore essential for the normal metabolism of glucose.

**Indications**

- Prior to administration of **50% dextrose** in patients with coma of unknown etiology, to prevent precipitation of Wernicke's encephalopathy.
- Known or suspected **thiamine deficiency** (beriberi).
- Chronic **alcoholism** and other states of general malnutrition.

**Contraindications**

None.

**Side Effects**

- Slight, transient **vasodilation** and **hypotension** after rapid IV administration.
- Overdosage may produce toxicity (weakness, dyspnea, respiratory failure).
- Rare **anaphylactic reactions.**

**How Supplied**

- Vials of 50 mg/ml.
- 1-ml, 5-ml, 10-ml, and 30-ml vials of 100 mg/ml.
- Tubex syringes of 100 mg.

**Administration and Dosage**

For coma, preceding the administration of 50% dextrose, give **50 mg slowly IV and 50 mg IM** (or, if there are signs of poor peripheral perfusion, give the entire 100 mg slowly IV).

**Incompatibility**

None of significance.

# Tissue Plasminogen Activator (rt-PA)

Activase

**Therapeutic Effects**

Enzyme that initiates the lysis of thrombi and thereby helps to reopen blocked coronary arteries in the acute phase of myocardial infarction.

**Indications**

Evolving **acute myocardial infarction** within the first 6 hours if inclusion criteria are met (see table).

**Contraindications**

- Active **internal bleeding** (e.g., peptic ulcer).
- Recent **stroke** or **intracranial surgery.**
- Severe, uncontrolled **hypertension.**
- Recent **trauma, surgery.**

**Side Effects**

- **Bleeding** tendency; fatal hemorrhage has occurred.
- **Fever.**
- **Hypotension.**
- **Nausea** and **vomiting.**
- Mild **allergic reactions.**

**How Supplied**

Powder in 20-mg and 50-mg vacuum-sealed vials packaged with diluent for reconstitution.

**Administration and Dosage**

Given by **intravenous infusion** through an **in-line filter.**

*Dosage:* Recommended dosage is 100 mg, of which

- **6 mg** is given as a **bolus over the first 1 to 2 minutes.**
- **54 mg** is then infused **over the first hour.**
- **20 mg** is infused over the **second hour.**
- **20 mg** is infused over the **third hour.**

**Incompatibility**

Do not administer to patients who have received **dextrans** or **anticoagulants.**

## *Criteria for Thrombolytic Therapy*

| Inclusion criteria | Exclusion criteria |
|---|---|
| Alert and able to give informed consent | Significant bleeding or known bleeding disorder |
| Age > 30 years | Stroke or transient ischemic attack |
| Chest pain for > 20 minutes and < 6 hours | History of gastrointestinal or genitourinary bleeding |
| Pain not relieved by sublingual nitroglycerin | Patient taking oral anticoagulant medication |
| Systolic BP > 80 and < 180 mm Hg | Insulin-dependent diabetes mellitus |
| Diastolic BP < 120 mm Hg | Terminal illness |
| Systolic pressure difference between the two arms < 20 mm Hg | Severe hypertension (systolic BP > 180 mm Hg, diastolic BP > 120 mm Hg) |
| ECG: S–T elevation of > 1 mm in two adjacent leads | Intravenous cannulas at noncompressible sites |

# Vecuronium Bromide

Norcuron

## Therapeutic Effects

Nondepolarizing neuromuscular blocking agent that competes for acetylcholine receptor sites at the motor end-plate. Provides effective **paralysis** of skeletal muscles within 3 minutes of administration. Recovery from paralysis requires 25 to 65 minutes, during which time the patient must be artificially ventilated.

## Indications

In the field, used principally to facilitate **crash intubation** in trauma victims with suspected head injuries, to prevent the increase in intracranial pressure that may be caused by succinylcholine when given alone.

## Contraindications

- **Operator not highly skilled** in emergency intubation.
- **Neuromuscular disease** (e.g., myasthenia gravis).
- Use with *caution* in patients with hepatic insufficiency.

## Side Effects

In some cases, the **effect** of the drug is **prolonged,** and controlled ventilation must be continued for some time.

## How Supplied

10-ml vials containing 10 mg of drug (1 mg/ml), with 10-ml prefilled syringes or 10-ml vials of diluent.
20-ml vials containing 20 mg of drug (1 mg/ml), to be diluted in normal saline or sterile water for injection.

## Vecuronium Bromide (continued)

**Administration and Dosage**

Given by **intravenous bolus injection.**

For rapid-sequence intubation in head trauma:

1. **Preoxygenate** the patient with 100% oxygen for 5 minutes.
2. Administer **vecuronium, 0.01 mg/kg IV.**
3. Administer *lidocaine,* 1.5 mg/kg IV.
4. Administer *fentanyl,* 3–5 μg/kg IV.
5. Wait 2 to 3 minutes. Continue preoxygenating with 100% oxygen.
6. Administer *thiopental,* 3–5 mg/kg IV (0.5–1.0 mg/kg if the patient is hypotensive).
7. Administer *succinylcholine,* 1.5 mg/kg.
8. Apply **cricoid pressure.**
9. **Intubate.**

**Incompatibility**

- Do not give **succinylcholine** *before* vecuronium.
- Do not give to patients receiving **aminoglycoside antibiotics** (neomycin, streptomycin, kanamycin, gentamicin); **tetracyclines, bacitracin, polymyxin B,** or **solistin,** all of which may prolong the neuromuscular blockade.
- Do not give to patients who are receiving **magnesium salts** for eclampsia.

# Verapamil

Isoptin, Calan, Ikakor

**Therapeutic Effects**

**Calcium channel blocker**; antagonizes the effects of calcium ion, thereby slowing sinoatrial node discharge and delaying conduction through the atrioventricular junction.

**Indications**

- Second-line drug for the treatment of **supraventricular tachycardias** that do not respond to vagal maneuvers or adenosine.
- To decrease the ventricular rate in some cases of **atrial flutter** and **atrial fibrillation.**

**Contraindications**

- **Cardiogenic shock** or **heart failure.**
- Sinus node disease ("**sick sinus syndrome**").
- **Hypotension** not due to tachyarrhythmia.
- Patient taking a **beta blocking drug** such as propranolol.
- **Wide-complex tachycardia.**

*Note:* Use with *caution* in elderly patients and in patients taking digitalis.

**Side Effects**

- **Hypotension.**
- Headache, **dizziness,** sweating.
- **AV** (atrioventricular) **block** or **bradycardia.**
- May cause **cardiac arrest.**
- May precipitate **heart failure** with pulmonary edema.

**How Supplied**

2-ml ampules and 4-ml vials containing 2.5 mg/ml.

## **Verapamil** (continued)

**Administration and Dosage**

Given by **slow intravenous injection** (over 1–2 minutes).

*Dosage:* **0.1 mg/kg** (usual adult dose, then, is 5–10 mg). May be repeated in 30 minutes.

**Incompatibility**

Do not use together with **beta blockers,** which may potentiate the effects of verapamil and precipitate heart failure.

| Generic Name<br>Trade Name |
|---|
| Therapeutic Effects |
| Indications |
| Contraindications |
| Side Effects |
| How Supplied |
| Administration and Dosage |
| Incompatibility |

| Generic Name<br>Trade Name |
| --- |
| Therapeutic Effects |
| Indications |
| Contraindications |
| Side Effects |
| How Supplied |
| Administration and Dosage |
| Incompatibility |

| Generic Name<br>Trade Name |
| --- |
| Therapeutic Effects |
| Indications |
| Contraindications |
| Side Effects |
| How Supplied |
| Administration and Dosage |
| Incompatibility |

| Generic Name<br>Trade Name |
| --- |
| Therapeutic Effects |
| Indications |
| Contraindications |
| Side Effects |
| How Supplied |
| Administration and Dosage |
| Incompatibility |

| Generic Name<br>Trade Name |
|---|
| Therapeutic Effects |
| Indications |
| Contraindications |
| Side Effects |
| How Supplied |
| Administration and Dosage |
| Incompatibility |

| Generic Name<br>Trade Name |
| --- |
| Therapeutic Effects |
| Indications |
| Contraindications |
| Side Effects |
| How Supplied |
| Administration and Dosage |
| Incompatibility |

| Generic Name<br>Trade Name |
| --- |
| Therapeutic Effects |
| Indications |
| Contraindications |
| Side Effects |
| How Supplied |
| Administration and Dosage |
| Incompatibility |

| Generic Name<br>Trade Name |
| --- |
| Therapeutic Effects |
| Indications |
| Contraindications |
| Side Effects |
| How Supplied |
| Administration and Dosage |
| Incompatibility |

# Index to Commonly Prescribed Drugs

This listing of prescription drugs is intended to help you identify the medications a patient may be taking at home and to make an educated guess as to the conditions for which the patient is being treated.

In the first index, the drugs are listed alphabetically by *trade name,* since that is the name often found on the label of prescription drugs. For each drug, there is an indication of its generic name, its general class (e.g., antihypertensive, antidepressant), and the condition(s) for which it is most commonly prescribed.

If you do not find the drug in the first index, it has probably been designated on the container by its *generic name.* In the second index, drugs are listed alphabetically by generic name, and the same information about the drugs is provided (trade name, class of drug, conditions for which it is most commonly prescribed).

# Index to Commonly Prescribed Drugs

## *Arranged by Trade Name*

| Trade name | Generic name | Class | Commonly prescribed for |
|---|---|---|---|
| Aarane | cromolyn | Mast cell inhibitor | Asthma |
| Actifed | pseudoephedrine | Beta sympathomimetic | Asthma |
| Adapin | doxepin | Tricyclic antidepressant | Depression |
| Aldactazide | hydrochlorothiazide + spironolactone | Diuretic | Hypertension |
| Aldactone | spironolactone | Diuretic | Hypertension |
| Aldoril | hydrochlorothiazide | Diuretic | Hypertension; CHF |
| Alupent | metaproterenol | Beta-2 sympathomimetic | Asthma |
| Amitril | amitriptyline | Tricyclic antidepressant | Depression |
| Amytal | amobarbital | Barbiturate | Sedation |
| Anaprox | naproxen | NSAID | Arthritis; pain; inflammation |
| Anhydron | cyclothiazide | Diuretic | Hypertension |
| Antabuse | disulfiram | Metabolic blocker | Alcoholism |
| Antivert | meclizine | Antihistamine | Vertigo |
| Apresoline | hydralazine | Vasodilator | Hypertension |
| Artane | trihexyphenidyl | Antispasmodic | Parkinson's disease |
| Asendin | amoxapine | Tricyclic antidepressant | Depression |
| Atarax | hydroxyzine | Antihistamine | Sedation |
| Ativan | lorazepam | Benzodiazepine tranquilizer | Anxiety; sleep |
| Atromid-S | clofibrate | Antilipidemic | To lower cholesterol |
| Atrovent | ipratropium | Bronchodilator | Asthma |
| Aventyl | nortriptyline | Tricyclic antidepressant | Depression |
| Azolid | phenylbutazone | Anti-inflammatory | Arthritis; inflammations |
| Bactrim | trimethoprim | Antibiotic | COPD; urinary tract infection |
| Beclovent | beclomethasone | Corticosteroid | Asthma |
| Beconase | beclomethasone | Corticosteroid | Asthma |
| Benadryl | diphenhydramine | Antihistamine | Allergies; hay fever |
| Benemid | probenecid | Uricosuric | Gout; hyperuricemia |
| Bentyl | dicyclomine | Anticholinergic | Nausea and vomiting |
| Blocadren | timolol maleate | Beta blocker | Angina; hypertension |
| Brethaire | terbutaline | Beta-2 sympathomimetic | Asthma |
| Brethine | terbutaline | Beta-2 sympathomimetic | Asthma |
| Bretylol | bretylium tosylate | Antiarrhythmic | Ventricular tachycardia |
| Bricanyl | terbutaline | Beta-2 sympathomimetic | Asthma |

# Index to Commonly Prescribed Drugs

## *Arranged by Trade Name* (continued)

| Trade name | Generic name | Class | Commonly prescribed for |
|---|---|---|---|
| Bronkosol | isoetharine | Bronchodilator | Asthma |
| Butazolidin | phenylbutazone | Anti-inflammatory | Arthritis; inflammations |
| Calan | verapamil | Calcium channel blocker | Coronary artery spasm; PSVT |
| Capastat | capreomycin | Antibiotic | Tuberculosis |
| Cardioquin | quinidine | Antiarrhythmic | Atrial/ventricular dysrhythmias |
| Cardizem | diltiazem | Calcium channel blocker | Angina |
| Catapres | clonidine | Vasodilator | Hypertension |
| Cibalith-S | lithium citrate | Anti-manic | Manic-depressive disorder |
| Clinoril | sulindac | NSAID | Arthritis |
| Cogentin | benztropine | Anticholinergic | Parkinson's disease |
| Compazine | prochlorperazine | Phenothiazine | Nausea; psychosis |
| Cordarone | amiodarone | Antiarrhythmic | Ventricular tachycardia |
| Corgard | nadolol | Beta blocker | Angina; hypertension |
| Corzide | nadolol | Beta blocker | Angina; hypertension |
| Coumadin | warfarin | Anticoagulant | Previous AMI; pulmonary embolism |
| Crystodigin | digitoxin | Cardiac glycoside | CHF; atrial dysrhythmias |
| Cyclospasmol | cyclandelate | Vasodilator | Nighttime leg cramps |
| Dalmane | flurazepam | Benzodiazepine tranquilizer | Sleep |
| Darvon | propoxyphene | Narcotic | Pain |
| Datril | acetaminophen | Analgesic/antipyretic | Pain; fever |
| Daxolin | loxapine | Antipsychotic | Psychosis |
| Demerol | meperidine | Narcotic | Pain |
| Demulen | ethinyl estradiol | Estrogen | Contraception |
| Depakene | valproic acid | Anticonvulsant | Seizures; neuropathic pain |
| Desyrel | trazodone | Antidepressant | Depression |
| DiaBeta | glyburide | Oral hypoglycemic | Diabetes |
| Diabinese | chlorpropamide | Oral hypoglycemic | Diabetes |
| Diamox | acetazolamide | Diuretic | Glaucoma |
| Dilantin | phenytoin | Anticonvulsant | Seizures |
| Dilaudid | hydromorphone | Narcotic | Pain |
| Diuril | chlorothiazide | Diuretic | Hypertension |

| Trade name | Generic name | Class | Commonly prescribed for |
|---|---|---|---|
| Dolobid | diflunisal | NSAID | Arthritis; inflammation |
| Donnatal | atropine + scopolamine + phenobarbital | Antispasmodic | Gastric or intestinal spasm |
| Doriden | glutethimide | Hypnotic | Sleep |
| Duraquin | quinidine | Antiarrhythmic | Atrial/ventricular dysrhythmias |
| Dyazide | hydrochlorothiazide | Diuretic | Hypertension; CHF |
| Dymelor | acetohexamide | Oral hypoglycemic | Diabetes |
| Dyrenium | triamterene | Diuretic | Hypertension |
| Edecrin | ethacrynic acid | Diuretic | Hypertension |
| Elavil | amitriptyline | Antidepressant | Depression; neuropathic pain |
| Elixophyllin | theophylline | Xanthine bronchodilator | Asthma; COPD |
| Endep | amitriptyline | Antidepressant | Depression; neuropathic pain |
| Enduron | methyclothiazide | Diuretic | CHF |
| Equanil | meprobamate | Barbiturate-like tranquilizer | Anxiety |
| Ery-Tab | erythromycin | Antibiotic | COPD; many infections |
| Esidrix | hydrochlorothiazide | Diuretic | Hypertension; CHF |
| Eskalith | lithium carbonate | Anti-manic | Manic-depressive disorder |
| Feldene | piroxicam | NSAID | Arthritis; inflammations |
| Feosol | ferrous sulfate | Iron | Iron-deficiency anemia |
| Fiorinal | aspirin + butalbital + caffeine | Analgesic | Pain |
| Flagyl | metronidazole | Antimicrobial | Infections |
| Flexeril | cyclobenzaprine | Smooth muscle relaxant | Muscle spasms |
| Gantanol | sulfamethoxazole | Antimicrobial sulfa drug | Urinary tract infection |
| Glucotrol | glipizide | Oral hypoglycemic | Diabetes |
| Halcion | triazolam | Benzodiazepine tranquilizer | Sleep |
| Haldol | haloperidol | Antipsychotic | Psychosis; nausea (low dose) |
| Humulin | insulin | Hormone | Diabetes |
| HydroDIURIL | hydrochlorothiazide | Diuretic | Hypertension; CHF |
| Hydropres | hydrochlorothiazide | Diuretic | Hypertension; CHF |
| Hygroton | chlorthalidone | Diuretic | Hypertension; CHF |
| Iletin | insulin | Hormone | Diabetes |
| Imavate | imipramine | Tricyclic antidepressant | Depression |

# Index to Commonly Prescribed Drugs

## *Arranged by Trade Name* (continued)

| Trade name | Generic name | Class | Commonly prescribed for |
|---|---|---|---|
| Inapsine | droperidol | Antipsychotic | Psychosis |
| Inderal | propranolol | Beta blocker | Angina; hypertension; tachyarrhythmias |
| Indocin | indomethacin | NSAID | Arthritis |
| Intal | cromolyn | Mast cell inhibitor | Asthma |
| Ismelin | guanethidine | Vasodilator | Hypertension |
| Isoptin | verapamil | Calcium channel blocker | Coronary artery spasm; PSVT |
| Isordil | isosorbide dinitrate | Nitroglycerin | Angina |
| Isosorb | isosorbide dinitrate | Nitroglycerin | Angina |
| Janimine | imipramine | Tricyclic antidepressant | Depression |
| Klonopin | clonazepam | CNS depressant | Seizures |
| K-Lyte | potassium chloride | Electrolyte | Potassium replacement |
| Lanoxin | digoxin | Cardiac glycoside | CHF; atrial dysrhythmias |
| Larodopa | levodopa | Dopamine precursor | Parkinson's disease |
| Lasix | furosemide | Diuretic | CHF; hypertension |
| Librium | chlordiazepoxide | Benzodiazepine tranquilizer | Anxiety |
| Lithane | lithium carbonate | Anti-manic | Manic-depressive disorder |
| Lithobid | lithium carbonate | Anti-manic | Manic-depressive disorder |
| Lithonate | lithium carbonate | Anti-manic | Manic-depressive disorder |
| Lomotil | diphenoxylate | Anticholinergic | Diarrhea |
| Lopressor | metoprolol | Beta blocker | Hypertension |
| Loxitane | loxapine | Antipsychotic | Psychosis |
| Ludiomil | maprotiline | Tricyclic antidepressant | Depression |
| Luminal | phenobarbital | Barbiturate | Seizures; sleep |
| Marax | ephedrine + theophylline | Bronchodilator | Asthma |
| Marplan | isocarboxazid | MAO inhibitor | Depression |
| Mellaril | thioridazine | Antipsychotic | Psychosis |
| Mesantoin | mephenytoin | Anticonvulsant | Seizures |
| Methahydrin | trichlormethiazide | Diuretic | Hypertension |
| Mexitil | mexiletine | Antiarrhythmic | Ventricular dysrhythmias |
| Micronase | glyburide | Oral hypoglycemic | Diabetes |
| Miltown | meprobamate | Barbiturate-like tranquilizer | Anxiety |
| Minipress | prazosin | Beta blocker | Hypertension |

| Trade name | Generic name | Class | Commonly prescribed for |
|---|---|---|---|
| Mixtard | insulin | Hormone | Diabetes |
| Moban | molindone | Antipsychotic | Psychosis |
| Motrin | ibuprofen | NSAID | Arthritis |
| Myambutol | ethambutol | Antibiotic | Tuberculosis |
| Mysoline | primidone | Anticonvulsant | Seizures |
| Nalfon | fenoprofen | NSAID | Arthritis |
| Naprosyn | naproxen | NSAID | Arthritis |
| Naqua | trichlormethiazide | Diuretic | Hypertension |
| Nardil | phenelzine | MAO inhibitor | Depression |
| Navane | thiothixene | Antipsychotic | Psychosis |
| Nembutal | pentobarbital | Barbiturate | Sleep |
| Nitro-Bid | nitroglycerin | Nitrate | Angina |
| Nitro-Dur | nitroglycerin | Nitrate | Angina |
| Nitrostat | nitroglycerin | Nitrate | Angina |
| Noctec | chloral hydrate | Hypnotic | Sleep |
| Noludar | methyprylon | Barbiturate-like hypnotic | Sleep |
| Norinyl | ethinyl estradiol | Estrogen | Contraception |
| Normodyne | labetalol | Beta blocker | Angina; hypertension |
| Norpace | disopryramide | Antiarrhythmic | PVCs |
| Norpramin | desipramine | Tricyclic antidepressant | Depression |
| Novolin | insulin | Hormone | Diabetes |
| Omnipen | ampicillin | Antibiotic | COPD; infections |
| Orap | pimozide | Antipsychotic | Psychosis |
| Oretic | hydrochlorothiazide | Diuretic | Hypertension; CHF |
| Orinase | tolbutamide | Oral hypoglycemic | Diabetes |
| Ortho-Novum | ethinyl estradiol | Estrogen | Contraception |
| Oxalid | oxyphenbutazone | NSAID | Arthritis |
| Pamelor | nortriptyline | Tricyclic antidepressant | Depression |
| Parnate | tranylcypromine | MAO inhibitor | Depression |
| Paxipam | halazepam | Benzodiazepine tranquilizer | Anxiety |
| Pepcid | famotidine | Antihistamine | Peptic ulcer disease |
| Percocet | oxycodone + acetaminophen | Narcotic | Pain |
| Percodan | oxycodone/aspirin | Narcotic | Pain |
| Periactin | cyproheptadine | Antihistamine | Colds; allergies |
| Permitil | fluphenazine | Antipsychotic | Psychosis |
| Persantine | dipyridamole | Antiarrhythmic | Ventricular dysrhythmias |
| Pertofrane | desipramine | Tricyclic antidepressant | Depression |
| Phenergan | promethazine | Antihistamine | Sedation |
| Placidyl | ethchlorvynol | Tranquilizer | Anxiety |
| Premarin | estrogens, conjugated | Hormone | Menopausal symptoms |
| Presamine | imipramine | Tricyclic antidepressant | Depression |
| Prilosec | omeprazole | Antihistamine | Peptic ulcer disease |
| Pro-Banthīne | propantheline | Anticholinergic | Spastic colon |

# Index to Commonly Prescribed Drugs

## *Arranged by Trade Name* (continued)

| Trade name | Generic name | Class | Commonly prescribed for |
|---|---|---|---|
| Procan | procainamide | Antiarrhythmic | Ventricular dysrhythmias |
| Procardia | nifedipine | Calcium channel blocker | Coronary artery spasm |
| Prolixin | fluphenazine | Antipsychotic | Psychosis |
| Proloid | thyroglobulin | Thyroid hormone | Hypothyroidism |
| Pronestyl | procainamide | Antiarrhythmic | Ventricular dysrhythmias |
| Proventil | albuterol | Beta-2 sympathomimetic | Asthma; COPD |
| Prozac | fluoxetine | Antidepressant | Depression |
| Quadrinal | theophylline | Xanthine bronchodilator | Asthma |
| Quibron | theophylline | Xanthine bronchodilator | Asthma |
| Quinaglute | quinidine | Antiarrhythmic | Atrial/ventricular dysrhythmias |
| Quinidex | quinidine | Antiarrhythmic | Atrial/ventricular dysrhythmias |
| Quinora | quinidine | Antiarrhythmic | Atrial/ventricular dysrhythmias |
| Regroton | reserpine + chlorthalidone | Vasodilator/ diuretic | Hypertension |
| Restoril | temazepam | Benzodiazepine tranquilizer | Sleep |
| Retrovir | zidovudine | Antiviral | AIDS |
| Rifadin | rifampin | Antibiotic | Tuberculosis |
| Rifamate | rifampin | Antibiotic | Tuberculosis |
| Ritalin | methylphenidate | CNS stimulant | Hyperactivity in children |
| Sandril | reserpine | Vasodilator | Hypertension |
| Seconal | secobarbital | Barbiturate | Sleep |
| Sectral | acebutolol | Beta blocker | Hypertension |
| Septra | trimethoprim | Antibiotic | COPD; urinary tract infection |
| Ser-Ap-Es | reserpine | Vasodilator | Hypertension |
| Serax | oxazepam | Benzodiazepine tranquilizer | Anxiety |
| Serentil | mesoridazine | Antipsychotic | Psychosis |
| Serpasil | reserpine | Vasodilator | Hypertension |
| Sinemet | levodopa | Dopamine precursor | Parkinson's disease |
| Sinequan | doxepin | Tricyclic antidepressant | Depression |
| SK-Pramine | imipramine | Tricyclic antidepressant | Depression |
| SK-65 | propoxyphene | Narcotic | Pain |
| Slo-Phyllin | theophylline | Xanthine bronchodilator | Asthma |
| Slow-K | potassium | Electrolyte | Potassium replacement |

| Trade name | Generic name | Class | Commonly prescribed for |
|---|---|---|---|
| Sorbitrate | isosorbide dinitrate | Nitroglycerin | Angina |
| Stelazine | trifluoperazine | Antipsychotic | Psychosis |
| Sudafed | pseudoephedrine | Beta sympathomimetic | Asthma; hay fever |
| Surmontil | trimipramine | Tricyclic antidepressant | Depression |
| Synthroid | levothyroxine | Thyroid hormone | Hypothyroidism |
| Tagamet | cimetidine | Antihistamine | Peptic ulcer disease |
| Talwin | pentazocine | Narcotic | Pain |
| Tambocor | flecainide | Antiarrhythmic | Ventricular dysrhythmias |
| Tapazole | methimazole | Thyroid inhibitor | Hyperthyroidism |
| Taractan | chlorprothixene | Antipsychotic | Psychosis |
| Tedral | theophylline | Xanthine bronchodilator | Asthma |
| Tegretol | carbamazepine | Anticonvulsant | Seizures; trigeminal neuralgia |
| Tenormin | atenolol | Beta blocker | Angina; hypertension; PSVT |
| Theo-Dur | theophylline | Xanthine bronchodilator | Asthma |
| Thorazine | chlorpromazine | Antipsychotic; antiemetic | Psychosis; vomiting |
| Tigan | trimethobenzamide | Antiemetic | Nausea and vomiting |
| Tofranil | imipramine | Tricyclic antidepressant | Depression |
| Tolectin | tolmetin | NSAID | Arthritis; pain |
| Tolinase | tolazamide | Oral hypoglycemic | Diabetes |
| Tonocard | tocainide | Antiarrhythmic | Ventricular dysrhythmias |
| Trandate | labetalol | Beta blocker | Angina; hypertension |
| Tranxene | clorazepate | Benzodiazepine tranquilizer | Anxiety |
| Trental | pentoxifylline | Antiviscosity agent | Intermittent claudication |
| Triavil | amitriptyline | Tricyclic antidepressant | Depression; neuropathic pain |
| Trilafon | perphenazine | Antipsychotic | Psychosis |
| Tylenol | acetaminophen | Analgesic/antipyretic | Pain; fever |
| Valium | diazepam | Benzodiazepine tranquilizer | Anxiety |
| Vancenase | beclomethasone | Corticosteroid | Asthma |
| Vanceril | beclomethasone | Corticosteroid | Asthma |
| Vaseretic | enalapril | Angiotensin inhibitor | Hypertension |
| Vasotec | enalapril | Angiotensin inhibitor | Hypertension |
| Velosulin | insulin | Hormone | Diabetes |
| Vesprin | triflupromazine | Antipsychotic | Psychosis |
| Visken | pindolol | Beta blocker | Angina; hypertension |

## *Arranged by Trade Name* (continued)

| Trade name | Generic name | Class | Commonly prescribed for |
|---|---|---|---|
| Vistaril | hydroxyzine | Antihistamine | Anxiety; nausea and vomiting; sleep |
| Wellbutrin | bupropion | Antidepressant | Depression |
| Xanax | alprazolam | Benzodiazepine tranquilizer | Anxiety |

AMI = acute myocardial infarction; CHF = congestive heart failure; CNS = central nervous system; COPD = chronic obstructive pulmonary disease; MAO = monoamine oxidase; NSAID = nonsteroidal anti-inflammatory drug; PVCs = premature ventricular contractions; PSVT = paroxysmal supraventricular tachycardia.

# Index to Commonly Prescribed Drugs

## *Arranged by Generic Name*

| Generic name | Trade name | Class | Commonly prescribed for |
|---|---|---|---|
| acebutolol | Sectral | Beta blocker | Hypertension |
| acetaminophen | Datril, Tylenol | Analgesic/antipyretic | Pain; fever |
| acetazolamide | Diamox | Diuretic | Glaucoma |
| acetohexamide | Dymelor | Oral hypoglycemic | Diabetes |
| albuterol | Proventil | Beta-2 sympathomimetic | Asthma; COPD |
| alprazolam | Xanax | Benzodiazepine tranquilizer | Anxiety |
| amiodarone | Cordarone | Antiarrhythmic | Ventricular tachycardia |
| amitriptyline | Amitril, Elavil, Endep, Triavil | Antidepressant | Depression; neuropathic pain |
| amobarbital | Amytal | Barbiturate | Sedation |
| amoxapine | Asendin | Tricyclic antidepressant | Depression |
| ampicillin | Omnipen | Antibiotic | COPD; infections |
| aspirin + butalbital + caffeine | Fiorinal | Analgesic | Pain |
| atenolol | Tenormin | Beta blocker | Angina; hypertension; PSVT |
| atropine + scopolamine + phenobarbital | Donnatal | Antispasmodic | Gastric or intestinal spasm |
| beclomethasone | Beclovent, Beconase, Vancenase, Vanceril | Corticosteroid | Asthma |
| benztropine | Cogentin | Anticholinergic | Parkinson's disease |
| bretylium tosylate | Bretylol | Antiarrhythmic | Ventricular tachycardia |
| bupropion | Wellbutrin | Antidepressant | Depression |
| capreomycin | Capastat | Antibiotic | Tuberculosis |
| carbamazepine | Tegretol | Anticonvulsant | Seizures; trigeminal neuralgia |
| chloral hydrate | Noctec | Hypnotic | Sleep |
| chlordiazepoxide | Librium | Benzodiazepine tranquilizer | Anxiety |
| chlorothiazide | Diuril | Diuretic | Hypertension |
| chlorpromazine | Thorazine | Antipsychotic; antiemetic | Psychosis; vomiting |
| chlorpropamide | Diabinese | Oral hypoglycemic | Diabetes |
| chlorprothixene | Taractan | Antipsychotic | Psychosis |
| chlorthalidone | Hygroton | Diuretic | Hypertension; CHF |
| cimetidine | Tagamet | Antihistamine | Peptic ulcer disease |

# Index to Commonly Prescribed Drugs

## *Arranged by Generic Name* (continued)

| Generic name | Trade name | Class | Commonly prescribed for |
|---|---|---|---|
| clofibrate | Atromid-S | Antilipidemic | To lower cholesterol |
| clonazepam | Klonopin | CNS depressant | Seizures |
| clonidine | Catapres | Vasodilator | Hypertension |
| clorazepate | Tranxene | Benzodiazepine tranquilizer | Anxiety |
| cromolyn | Aarane, Intal | Mast cell inhibitor | Asthma |
| cyclandelate | Cyclospasmol | Vasodilator | Nighttime leg cramps |
| cyclobenzaprine | Flexeril | Smooth muscle relaxant | Muscle spasms |
| cyclothiazide | Anhydron | Diuretic | Hypertension |
| cyproheptadine | Periactin | Antihistamine | Colds; allergies |
| desipramine | Norpramin, Pertofrane | Tricyclic antidepressant | Depression |
| diazepam | Valium | Benzodiazepine tranquilizer | Anxiety |
| dicyclomine | Bentyl | Anticholinergic | Nausea and vomiting |
| diflunisal | Dolobid | NSAID | Arthritis; inflammation |
| digitoxin | Crystodigin | Cardiac glycoside | CHF; atrial dysrhythmias |
| digoxin | Lanoxin | Cardiac glycoside | CHF; atrial dysrhythmias |
| diltiazem | Cardizem | Calcium channel blocker | Angina |
| diphenhydramine | Benadryl | Antihistamine | Allergies; hay fever |
| diphenoxylate | Lomotil | Anticholinergic | Diarrhea |
| dipyridamole | Persantine | Antiarrhythmic | Ventricular dysrhythmias |
| disopyramide | Norpace | Antiarrhythmic | PVCs |
| disulfiram | Antabuse | Metabolic blocker | Alcoholism |
| doxepin | Adapin, Sinequan | Tricyclic antidepressant | Depression |
| droperidol | Inapsine | Antipsychotic | Psychosis |
| enalapril | Vaseretic, Vasotec | Angiotensin inhibitor | Hypertension |
| ephedrine + theophylline | Marax | Bronchodilator | Asthma |
| erythromycin | Ery-Tab | Antibiotic | COPD; many infections |
| estrogens, conjugated | Premarin | Hormone | Menopausal symptoms |
| ethacrynic acid | Edecrin | Diuretic | Hypertension |
| ethambutol | Myambutol | Antibiotic | Tuberculosis |
| ethchlorvynol | Placidyl | Tranquilizer | Anxiety |
| ethinyl estradiol | Demulen, Norinyl, Ortho-Novum | Estrogen | Contraception |

| Generic name | Trade name | Class | Commonly prescribed for |
|---|---|---|---|
| famotidine | Pepcid | Antihistamine | Peptic ulcer disease |
| fenoprofen | Nalfon | NSAID | Arthritis |
| ferrous sulfate | Feosol | Iron | Iron-deficiency anemia |
| flecainide | Tambocor | Antiarrhythmic | Ventricular dysrhythmias |
| fluoxetine | Prozac | Antidepressant | Depression |
| fluphenazine | Permitil, Prolixin | Antipsychotic | Psychosis |
| flurazepam | Dalmane | Benzodiazepine tranquilizer | Sleep |
| furosemide | Lasix | Diuretic | CHF; hypertension |
| glipizide | Glucotrol | Oral hypoglycemia | Diabetes |
| glutethimide | Doriden | Hypnotic | Sleep |
| glyburide | DiaBeta, Micronase | Oral hypoglycemic | Diabetes |
| guanethidine | Ismelin | Vasodilator | Hypertension |
| halazepam | Paxipam | Benzodiazepine tranquilizer | Anxiety |
| haloperidol | Haldol | Antipsychotic | Psychosis; nausea (low dose) |
| hydralazine | Apresoline | Vasodilator | Hypertension |
| hydrochlorothiazide | Aldoril, Dyazide, Esidrix, HydroDIURIL, Hydropres, Oretic | Diuretic | Hypertension; CHF |
| hydrochlorothiazide + spironolactone | Aldactazide | Diuretic | Hypertension |
| hydromorphone | Dilaudid | Narcotic | Pain |
| hydroxyzine | Atarax, Vistaril | Antihistamine | Sedation; nausea/vomiting |
| ibuprofen | Motrin | NSAID | Arthritis |
| imipramine | Imavate, Janimine, Presamine, Sk-Pramine, Tofranil | Tricyclic antidepressant | Depression |
| indomethacin | Indocin | NSAID | Arthritis |
| insulin | Humulin, Iletin, Mixtard, Novolin, Velosulin | Hormone | Diabetes |
| ipratropium | Atrovent | Bronchodilator | Asthma |
| isocarboxazid | Marplan | MAO inhibitor | Depression |
| isoetharine | Bronkosol | Bronchodilator | Asthma |
| isosorbide dinitrate | Isordil, Isosorb, Sorbitrate | Nitroglycerin | Angina |
| labetalol | Normodyne, Trandate | Beta blocker | Angina; hypertension |
| levodopa | Larodopa, Sinemet | Dopamine precursor | Parkinson's disease |
| levothyroxine | Synthroid | Thyroid hormone | Hypothyroidism |

# Index to Commonly Prescribed Drugs

## *Arranged by Generic Name* (continued)

| Generic name | Trade name | Class | Commonly prescribed for |
|---|---|---|---|
| lithium carbonate | Eskalith, Lithane, Lithobid, Lithonate | Anti-manic | Manic-depressive disorder |
| lithium citrate | Cibalith-S | Anti-manic | Manic-depressive disorder |
| lorazepam | Ativan | Benzodiazepine tranquilizer | Anxiety; sleep |
| loxapine | Daxolin, Loxitane | Antipsychotic | Psychosis |
| maprotiline | Ludiomil | Tricyclic anti-depressant | Depression |
| meclizine | Antivert | Antihistamine | Vertigo |
| meperidine | Demerol | Narcotic | Pain |
| mephenytoin | Mesantoin | Anticonvulsant | Seizures |
| meprobamate | Equanil, Miltown | Barbiturate-like tranquilizer | Anxiety |
| mesoridazine | Serentil | Antipsychotic | Psychosis |
| metaproterenol | Alupent | Beta-2 sympatho-mimetic | Asthma |
| methimazole | Tapazole | Thyroid inhibitor | Hyperthyroidism |
| methyclothiazide | Enduron | Diuretic | CHF |
| methylphenidate | Ritalin | CNS stimulant | Hyperactivity in children |
| methyprylon | Noludar | Barbiturate-like hypnotic | Sleep |
| metoprolol | Lopressor | Beta blocker | Hypertension |
| metronidazole | Flagyl | Antimicrobial | Infections |
| mexiletine | Mexitil | Antiarrhythmic | Ventricular dys-rhythmias |
| molindone | Moban | Antipsychotic | Psychosis |
| nadolol | Corgard, Corzide | Beta blocker | Angina; hyperten-sion |
| naproxen | Anaprox, Naprosyn | NSAID | Arthritis; pain; in-flammation |
| nifedipine | Procardia | Calcium channel blocker | Coronary artery spasm |
| nitroglycerin | Nitro-Bid, Nitro-Dur, Nitrostat | Nitrate | Angina |
| nortriptyline | Aventyl, Pamelor | Tricyclic anti-depressant | Depression |
| omeprazole | Prilosec | Antihistamine | Peptic ulcer disease |
| oxazepam | Serax | Benzodiazepine tranquilizer | Anxiety |
| oxycodone + acet-aminophen | Percocet | Narcotic | Pain |
| oxycodone/aspirin | Percodan | Narcotic | Pain |
| oxyphenbutazone | Oxalid | NSAID | Arthritis |
| pentazocine | Talwin | Narcotic | Pain |

| Generic name | Trade name | Class | Commonly prescribed for |
|---|---|---|---|
| pentobarbital | Nembutal | Barbiturate | Sleep |
| pentoxifylline | Trental | Antiviscosity agent | Intermittent claudication |
| perphenazine | Trilafon | Antipsychotic | Psychosis |
| phenelzine | Nardil | MAO inhibitor | Depression |
| phenobarbital | Luminal | Barbiturate | Seizures; sleep |
| phenylbutazone | Azolid, Butazolidin | Anti-inflammatory | Arthritis; inflammations |
| phenytoin | Dilantin | Anticonvulsant | Seizures |
| pimozide | Orap | Antipsychotic | Psychosis |
| pindolol | Visken | Beta blocker | Angina; hypertension |
| piroxicam | Feldene | NSAID | Arthritis; inflammations |
| potassium | Slow-K | Electrolyte | Potassium replacement |
| potassium chloride | K-Lyte | Electrolyte | Potassium replacement |
| prazosin | Minipress | Beta blocker | Hypertension |
| primidone | Mysoline | Anticonvulsant | Seizures |
| probenecid | Benemid | Uricosuric | Gout; hyperuricemia |
| procainamide | Procan, Pronestyl | Antiarrhythmic | Ventricular dysrhythmias |
| prochlorperazine | Compazine | Phenothiazine | Nausea; psychosis |
| promethazine | Phenergan | Antihistamine | Sedation |
| propantheline | Pro-Banthīne | Anticholinergic | Spastic colon |
| propoxyphene | Darvon-N, Sk-65 | Narcotic | Pain |
| propranolol | Inderal | Beta blocker | Angina; hypertension; tachyarrythmias |
| pseudoephedrine | Actifed, Sudafed | Beta sympathomimetic | Asthma; hay fever |
| quinidine | Cardioquin, Duraquin, Quinaglute, Quinidex, Quinora | Antiarrhythmic | Atrial/ventricular dysrhythmias |
| reserpine | Sandril, Ser-Ap-Es, Serpasil | Vasodilator | Hypertension |
| reserpine + chlorthalidone | Regroton | Vasodilator/ diuretic | Hypertension |
| rifampin | Rifadin, Rifamate | Antibiotic | Tuberculosis |
| secobarbital | Seconal | Barbiturate | Sleep |
| spironolactone | Aldactone | Diuretic | Hypertension |
| sulfamethoxazole | Gantanol | Antimicrobial sulfa drug | Urinary tract infection |
| sulindac | Clinoril | NSAID | Arthritis |
| temazepam | Restoril | Benzodiazepine tranquilizer | Sleep |
| terbutaline | Brethaire, Brethine, Bricanyl | Beta-2 sympathomimetic | Asthma |

# Index to Commonly Prescribed Drugs

## *Arranged by Generic Name* (continued)

| Generic name | Trade name | Class | Commonly prescribed for |
|---|---|---|---|
| theophylline | Elixophyllin, Quadrinal, Quibron, Slo-Phyllin, Tedral, Theo-Dur | Xanthine bronchodilator | Asthma; COPD |
| thioridazine | Mellaril | Antipsychotic | Psychosis |
| thiothixene | Navane | Antipsychotic | Psychosis |
| thyroglobulin | Proloid | Thyroid hormone | Hypothyroidism |
| timolol maleate | Blocadren | Beta blocker | Angina; hypertension |
| tocainide | Tonocard | Antiarrhythmic | Ventricular dysrhythmias |
| tolazamide | Tolinase | Oral hypoglycemic | Diabetes |
| tolbutamide | Orinase | Oral hypoglycemic | Diabetes |
| tolmetin | Tolectin | NSAID | Arthritis; pain |
| tranylcypromine | Parnate | MAO inhibitor | Depression |
| trazodone | Desyrel | Antidepressant | Depression |
| triamterene | Dyrenium | Diuretic | Hypertension |
| triazolam | Halcion | Benzodiazepine tranquilizer | Sleep |
| trichlormethiazide | Methahydrin, Naqua | Diuretic | Hypertension |
| trifluoperazine | Stelazine | Antipsychotic | Psychosis |
| triflupromazine | Vesprin | Antipsychotic | Psychosis |
| trihexyphenidyl | Artane | Antispasmodic | Parkinson's disease |
| trimethobenzamide | Tigan | Antiemetic | Nausea and vomiting |
| trimethoprim | Bactrim, Septra | Antibiotic | COPD; urinary tract infection |
| trimipramine | Surmontil | Tricyclic antidepressant | Depression |
| valproic acid | Depakene | Anticonvulsant | Seizures; neuropathic pain |
| verapamil | Calan, Isoptin | Calcium channel blocker | Coronary artery spasm; PSVT |
| warfarin | Coumadin | Anticoagulant | Previous AMI; pulmonary embolism |
| zidovudine | Retrovir | Antiviral | AIDS |

AMI = acute myocardial infarction; CHF = congestive heart failure; CNS = central nervous system; COPD = chronic obstructive pulmonary disease; MAO = monoamine oxidase; NSAID = nonsteroidal anti-inflammatory drug; PVCs = premature ventricular contractions; PSVT = paroxysmal supraventricular tachycardia.

# Index